JEANNE E. BLUMBERG
ELEANOR E. DRUMMOND

Nursing Care of the Long-Term Patient

SECOND EDITION

**NURSING CARE OF THE
LONG-TERM PATIENT**

Nursing Care of the Long-Term Patient

Second Edition

JEANNE E. BLUMBERG
R.N., P.H.N., M.S.
*Formerly Visiting
Professor of Public
Health Nursing,
School of Nursing,
Hacettepe University,
Ankara, Turkey*

ELEANOR E. DRUMMOND
R.N., P.H.N., Ed.D.
*Professor of Nursing,
School of Nursing,
Boston University*

SPRINGER PUBLISHING COMPANY, INC.
New York

First Edition, 1963
Second Edition
   First Printing, May, 1971
   Second Printing, July, 1971

Copyright © 1971

Springer Publishing Company, Inc.
200 Park Avenue South, New York, New York 10003

All rights reserved

Library of Congress Catalog Card Number: 78-130686

Standard Book Number 0-8261-0612-9
Printed in the U.S.A.

PREFACE TO THE SECOND EDITION

The basic essentials of the nursing care of the long-term patient were set forth in the original edition of this book. They have not changed. However, many nursing, medical, technical and societal discoveries and innovations have prompted this revision.

In Chapter I a suggested framework, or "model", is added, upon which the nurse can organize existing knowledges, skills, and techniques into an understandable, workable whole.

The succeeding chapters were reorganized in sequence in accordance with the model. Many of the chapters were completely rewritten. Some were expanded to include current care; some were condensed to delete outdated material.

The focus of this book remains the same: excellence of nursing care for patients with long-term illnesses.

March 1971

JEANNE E. BLUMBERG
ELEANOR E. DRUMMOND

PREFACE TO
THE FIRST EDITION

This book is written for every nurse interested in excellence of care for patients who have long-term illnesses. It was developed for two main purposes. One is to propose a way of looking at patient care in long-term illness, a way which is based upon reality and tempered with imagination; the other is to organize existing knowledge that is basic to the art of nursing long-term patients into an understandable whole.

This book endeavors to develop an attitude toward the long-term patient which is conducive to the excellence of his nursing care. Each chapter projects a specific attitude toward the long-term patient and his family which contributes to a therapeutic relationship between the nurse and the patient. The book as a whole springs from the enthusiasm and satisfactions, felt by each of us, from caring for the long-term patient. We hope the readers will discover the wonders derived from exploring and solving with the patient many of his nursing problems. This is the first purpose of our book.

Attitudes toward nursing the long-term patient are extremely important, but they are only one aspect of the art of nursing. They cannot substitute for the identification, organization, execution, and evaluation of nursing care which is built upon an understanding of current knowledge of disease entities, drugs, physiology, human behavior, and related disciplines. The excellence of nursing is developed by the nurse through continual effort, mastery of technical skills and procedures, and grasp and retention of subject matter. Methods for developing manual skills, delineation of procedures, guides for evaluation, and guides for the use of principles abound in the nursing literature. From these, the reader is expected to obtain all these essentials of nursing care. Turning to this book, the reader will find subject matter requisite to the art of nursing long-term patients. To organize this material is the second purpose of our book.

Two problems face the nurse attempting to grasp and use the information relating to long-term illness. One problem is that of quantity. The wealth of printed material available to the nurse is valuable only when she applies the content to her own situation and to the development of her own art of nursing. This book is not an exhaustive condensation of current theories and facts. It is planned as a point of reference from which the nurse may proceed into nursing and non-nursing literature. Some specific information, techniques, and skills have been included in each chapter. The illustrations of the application of the materials in selected nursing situations have been taken from the past experience of both of us.

The second, related problem is that of organizing, systematizing, and classifying information. In solving this problem, we have used eight key concepts of direct nursing care of the long-term patient and his family. Professional nursing other than that practiced in a continuous nurse-patient and nurse-family relation is not included in the key concepts nor contained in the book. Chapter 1 shows the scope of the chronic disease problem and introduces the key concepts. The succeeding Chapters (2 through 9) each present one key concept and the components of patient care which form that concept. The components tend to be exhaustive but are not mutually exclusive. This organization of subject matter, developed by one of us, Dr. Drummond, in a three-year study, has been used in teaching long-term illness nursing.

Organization, analysis, and classification of knowledge is essential but is not enough. Therefore, Chapters 10 and 11 illustrate the synthesis of the key concepts of long-term illness nursing in actual situations.

Since key concepts epitomize common features of a large number of ideas, we believe this book will assist the nurse, within her particular frame of reference, to grasp the broad knowledge of long-term illness nursing. We hope that she will find a stimulation to develop excellence in the care of long-term patients.

This book was conceived and implemented as a cooperative project. Although both of us assume overall responsibility for the entire book, chapters 1, 4, 5, 6, and 9 were primarily Dr. Drummond's responsibility; chapters 2, 3, 7, and 8 were primarily Mrs. Blumberg's; chapters 10 and 11 were joint responsibilities.

March 1963

J. E. B.
E. E. D.

ACKNOWLEDGMENTS

For arrangements made with various publishing houses and authors, whereby certain copyrighted material was permitted to be reprinted, and for the courtesy extended by them, acknowledgments are gratefully made:

to Joseph Fletcher, Professor of Christian Ethics, Episcopal Theological School, Cambridge, Massachusetts, for the quotation from his article "The Patient's Right to Die," published in *Harper's Magazine;*

to Hildegard E. Peplau and G. P. Putnam's Sons, for definitions of certain nurse-patient relationships in her book "Interpersonal Relations in Nursing;"

to the Blakiston Div., McGraw-Hill Book Co., Inc., for the use, in slightly modified form, of four case studies in "Death and the Curriculum," by the authors, published in *The Journal of Nursing Education.*

Full bibliographic data will be found in the chapters containing the reprinted material.

CONTENTS

CHAPTER

1 A Model for Nursing Care 1
2 Observation 15
3 Physical Care 28
4 Emotional Support 40
5 Treatment 57
6 Teaching 67
7 Counseling 78
8 Economics 87
9 Complex Correlations 95
10 Death, The Inevitable: An Approach 107
11 A Case Study: A Model for Nursing Care 125

1 A MODEL FOR NURSING CARE

The health needs of the United States are shifting. There is an increase in the number of patients with illnesses requiring care over an extended period of time. These are the "long-term patients." There are no age limitations for these patients, since long-term illness can occur in any age group. The diabetic child, the middle-aged patient with a new ileostomy, the retired businessman recovering from a cerebral-vascular incident—each needs guidance in adapting to new living patterns as he learns to cope with his medical problems. Even these few examples indicate the challenging type of nursing care necessary to help bring about an optimal adaptation by the patient to the disruption in his life caused by ill health.

Nursing education is, fortunately, moving away from the disease-centered approach. It is now recognized that, while a knowledge of specific changes in pathology, structure, and function is important in nursing, this alone is not enough if the nurse is to give the quality of care needed by the long-term patient.

The following definitions are given to clarify terms in this book:

Long-term patients are "those persons suffering from chronic disease or impairments who require a prolonged period of care, that is, who are likely to need or who have received care for a continuous period of at least 30 days in a general hospital, or care for a continuous period of more than three months in another institution or at home, such care to include medical supervision and/or assistance in achieving a higher level of self-care and independence.[1]"

Long-term patients, regardless of the disease causing the disability, have certain common needs. In addition to nursing care and supervision,[2] they may need financial assistance, rehabilitation services,[3] and help with emotional disturbances resulting from prolonged hospitalization and the devaluating attitudes of the public toward patients with extended illness.[4]

The long-term patient is not necessarily the same as a person with a chronic disease, and not all persons with a chronic disease are long-term patients. Chronic disease was defined by the Commission on Chronic Illness in 1951 as follows:

Chronic disease comprises all impairments or deviations from the normal which have one or more of the following:

> are permanent
> leave residual disability
> are caused by non-reversible pathological alteration
> require special training of the patient for rehabilitation
> may be expected to require a long period of supervision, observation or care.[5]

The element of time makes a profound difference in the relationship between nurse and long-term patient. Although neglect of the subtleties of care, insensitivity to unspoken needs, or avoidance of planning for discharge may be tolerated by the patient during a short crisis period, when the nurse-patient relationship lasts for at least 30 days in the hospital or three months at home, quality of communication and care is essential if the nurse expects to be therapeutic. The nurse needs a holistic approach to the patient so that all the important aspects of care are planned and implemented.

We wish to present a model of nursing care. This model comprises eight parts or components. Each will be discussed in detail in the following chapters, and each focuses on the one-to-one relationship of the nurse with a patient who has nursing needs that extend over time. The model is designed to be useful to all areas of nursing, but the focus is on the challenges and needs presented by the long-term patient.

As an aid to developing a synthesis of nursing knowledge, a structure is needed in which to place the separate parts. Each part is important to the whole. Model building provides a structure for the fitting of separate knowledges and skills of nursing into a reasonable whole. Model building is also a vital step in the development of nursing theory.[6] What, then, is a model?

A model is a description or analogy used to help visualize something (e.g., an atom) that cannot be directly observed. The term "model" should not be confused with the currently used term "module," which is an assembly of wired electronic components.

The model presented here is visualized as having eight interlocking parts. Others in the field of nursing may visualize the totality of patient care in other forms or in a different number of parts. However, the totality of patient care is not complete if any one of our eight components is discarded. There will be times in the giving of nursing care that one or more of the components will have a higher priority, but the nursing needs of the patient cannot be met without consideration of all of the components.

To build the model we will first look at the patient and what he brings to the nurse-patient relationship. Visualize the patient as a cone on a base of life experiences. He is what he is today with his illness and health needs and cannot be separated from his previous life experiences as they have a profound influence on his health needs and/or on his ability to recover.

A part of the base that both influences nursing care and contributes to our understanding of the patient is the economics related to the current disability. Another part comprises social and ethnic factors that contribute to the precipitation or maintenance of certain disease entities the patient presents to the nursing profession for care. Social and ethnic factors are called *complex correlations* for want of a better term to designate certain patterns of disease that are known to occur.

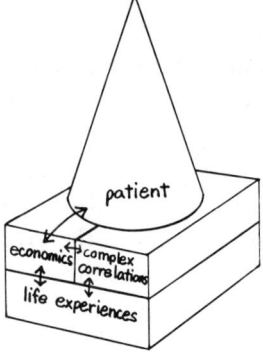

A MODEL FOR NURSING CARE

Next, let us look at the specific skills of nursing—observation, physical care, emotional support, treatment, teaching, and counseling. These are the skill components that combine knowledge with learned behaviors such as manual dexterity and listening. The skill components can be viewed as concentric circles that fit over and around the patient.

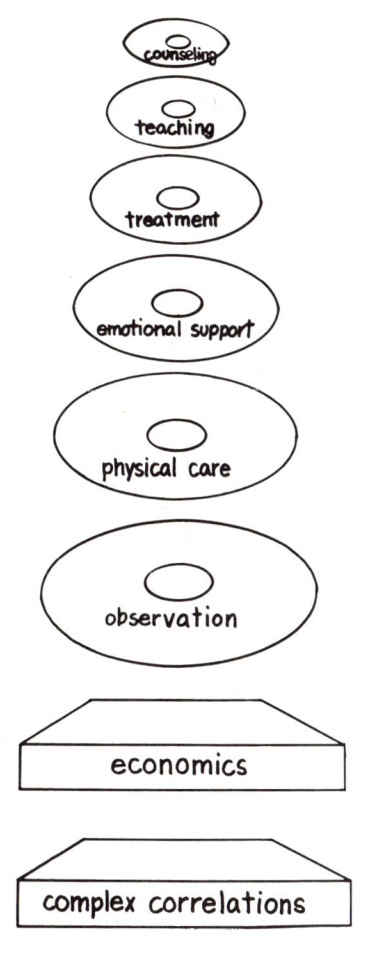

- counseling
- teaching
- treatment
- emotional support
- physical care
- observation
- economics
- complex correlations

When fitted together as a totality, the model has the following interesting shape.

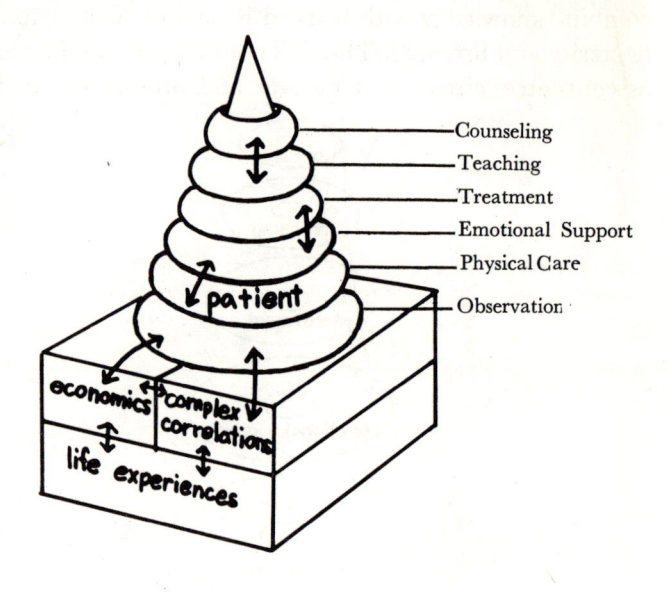

- Counseling
- Teaching
- Treatment
- Emotional Support
- Physical Care
- Observation

(patient; economics, complex correlations, life experiences)

The system is interlocking, as the arrows indicate, and includes all aspects of the nurse-patient relationship. Although the parts are divided for identification, the model is only complete with all of the proposed parts. The whole may be divided or visualized in different patterns, but any pattern should consider all of the six skill components, the two knowledge components, and the patient as a unique being with specific nursing needs.

It should be noted that the model was constructed with the patient in the center. Any model or any development of nursing theory must consider the patient as an essential unit of the structure.[7] The interlocking nature of the model is also vital.[8] "Nursing requires the recognition of the inseparability and interdependence of many factors."[9] The consideration of all components in combination helps the nurse attain a holistic approach to patient care. The combination is more than the sum of the individual components of care.

The concentric circles of the skill components are built on each other with the idea that observation is basic to all the other skills, that emotional support is built on physical care, etc. The ascending order of the skill components moves from closeness to increasing distance from physical contact. For example, in counseling the nurse may be physically removed from the patient as she discusses the patient's problems with representatives of the other health disciplines.

This model has been useful in teaching baccalaureate students during the past ten years. It is, also, adaptable for in-service education to help the nurse practitioner look at nursing as a unity and not simply as a series of unrelated tasks to be completed.

Having stated that nursing is a whole, we now introduce the nursing care components that will be developed in the following chapters.

Observation

Observation is dependent on the skill of the observer. But first there has to be an observer on the spot. Subtle changes cannot be observed if the time spent with the patient is short, and even marked changes cannot be observed from the chair in the nurses' station.

Observation includes the full use of all the physical senses and the proverbial "sixth sense." The nurse must hear, see, smell, taste, and feel—physically and with intuition. The purpose of observation is to gather information upon which to make judgments. The more information there is, the sounder the judgment can be and the clearer the report to the physician and others. Observation based on close contact with the patient is vital in making an accurate nursing care plan.

Full use of all the nurse's faculties is all the more necessary because many new therapies are known to be toxic. Thus, the nurse must use her observation not only for recognition of disease symptoms but also for the discovery and reporting of known and unknown (or previously unreported) adverse reactions to therapy.

Physical care

The close personal interaction that is a necessary part of giving physical care to the patient is basic to the other nursing components. The decrease of distance—physical, emotional and social—between the nurse and patient should be the means to the eventual rehabilitation of the patient.

Current practice in medical care, because of its increased armamentarium of drugs and techniques, tends to stress early independence of the patient by early ambulation, early self-care, and early discharge from the hospital. We should not generalize, however. By definition, the long-term patient remains in a hospital for 30 days or longer and needs care at home for three months or longer.

An important activity of the nurse, while helping the patient to independence, is to care for those personal needs the patient cannot perform by himself, such as combing the hair, cleaning and trimming the nails, turning and positioning in bed. These activities are usually classified as "unchallenging," but their mastery may be decisive in determining the eventual rehabilitation of the patient.

Emotional support

To give emotional support to patients, the nurse needs to understand her own emotional life. Her emotions may be thought of as a tool to be used in shaping the nurse-patient relationship. But no tool can be properly and effectively used unless its capabilities and functions are understood.

How the nurse feels, how she reacts to people and situations, how sensitive she is to the verbal and non-verbal communications of the patient must all be brought to the conscious level of the nurse's understanding. The nurse at a conscious level can then use, change, and adapt her emotional life so that it becomes a therapeutic tool in the nurse-patient interaction.

The nurse must understand not only herself but the patient as well—what the impact of long-term illness on the patient will be and how he may react to it emotionally. Loss is a common occurrence in long-term illness: loss of function, loss of a part of the body, loss of a comfortable or stabilized body image, loss of economic or personal independence. Loss, whether real or threatened, is usually followed by a period of mourning or grief. The nurse who expects grief after loss is better prepared to help the patient while he is grieving and when he is trying to find a way out of the grief period.

Treatment

The presence of several diseases within one person is common, particularly in the long-term patient. Besides the specific diseases, there is social and emotional displacement of the patient. The physician may experience difficulty in treating the patient because of these complexities.

The nurse, on her part, needs to know therapeutic and diagnostic procedures, dosage and administration of medications, and must have technical skill in manipulation of equipment. The knowledge and skill needed differs with each disease and the theory held on the treatment of that disease. Also, a treatment that may be in use in one part of the country may not be followed in another. The efforts of the drug houses and manufacturers of apparatus, and the varied aims of research contribute further to the fluidity of the treatment pattern for the long-term patient.

The ability of the nurse to keep up with current treatment patterns is more important than knowledge of isolated or dated facts. Without continual reading she cannot possibly keep informed about what is current and valuable in the complex treatment of the long-term patient. The nurse also must develop a system of accumulating her knowledge of treatments, for example by keeping a list or card file of new drugs. Activities like these reinforce learning and make it more available for application in practice.

Teaching the patient

The things nurses say, how they answer the patient's questions, the things they leave unsaid, how they do the ordered treatments, how they introduce new medications, all these are teaching activities of the nurse. When two people come together, *some* learning and therefore some teaching will occur. The plea is that the teaching have purpose and direction, and that the learning the patient does be of value to him—so that he will know more about his illness or develop skills in caring for himself or give himself the treatments ordered by his physician.

Teaching by the nurse is of major importance in long-term illness nursing. It must be based on accurate infor-

A MODEL FOR NURSING CARE

mation and adapted to the patient's ability to learn. Generally, the patient with a long-term illness has to accept more responsibility for treatments and medications continued after discharge from the hospital than other patients. Therefore, the nurse needs to focus her teaching not only on what *she is doing* in a treatment but also on how *the patient can adapt* the activity to his manual skills and home situation.

Counseling and working with others

As medical treatment becomes more complex, as social agencies develop and expand, the cooperation between the health and social agencies becomes more important. Too frequently, the patient and his family are lost in the multiplicity of services. As more members are added to the health team to solve the complex social, physical, and psychological problems of the long-term patient, each member seems to do less or assume less responsibility for the patient—a trend not conducive to producing a solution of the patient's problems.

Just as a nurse must work with members of the health team, so she must work with members of the patient's family. An understanding of the family's social, ethnic, and religious life is necessary if the nurse is to help the family plan the adaptation of treatments and living arrangements to the home situation. Inadequate planning with the family frequently upsets the continuity of care as the patient moves from the hospital to his home.

Economics of disability

Long-term illness and poverty go hand in hand in our country. This is a cliché, but it must be remembered by the nurse who aims at giving complete nursing care to the long-term patient and his family. The nurse has responsibility for the economic aspect of nursing care.

The cost of medical care today is increasing. In long-term illness, the need for continual medical and nursing supervision is extended over a long period, in many instances for the rest of the patient's lifetime. While the medical costs to the patient and his family increase, his employment opportunities and income potential generally decrease. It is almost impossible in our country to secure adequate financial protection against long-term illness before it occurs.

The nurse must understand and be able to counsel the patient and his family about their financial situation, the employment potential of the patient and family, the cost of medical supervision, general household expenses, hospital charges, and cost of equipment. The nurse must also be aware of, and point out, outside sources of financial aid available to patients and families, such as medicaid, Old Age Survivor's Insurance, Workman's Compensation, the categorical aids of the Bureau of Public Assistance, and the many philanthropic institutions. Many times it is up to the nurse to take the initiative for referring patients to such agencies and organizations because she is the only professional worker in day-to-day contact with the patient and his family.

The economic component of nursing intervention may include responsibility for conserving costly equipment or for improvising equipment in the home situations. Diet planning and income budgeting often become nursing responsibilities. When these tasks are skillfully handled, they will alleviate family difficulties, improve the patient's state of health, and contribute to his recovery.

A MODEL FOR NURSING CARE

Complex correlations

Not so long ago it used to be enough for the nurse to know the textbook picture of a disease and then plan her nursing care from this base. Yet it is unrealistic to consider a disease as existing separately and alone. The germ theory has been of great help in the control of many diseases, but it has also clouded the importance of other factors in the etiology and maintenance of disease. The number one health problem in the United States today is chronic disease, including arthritis, cancer, heart disease, and diabetes. These are our current leading causes of death. They have no known etiological agent.

A new body of knowledge has become important for the nurse, namely the recognition of the complex correlations between the patient, his personality, his family background, other diseases, and non-specific stress. The disease, the host, the social, ethnic, religious, and physical environment must be looked upon as one intricate complex. Knowledge of the relationships that exist between the parts is what guides the nurse to plan her care of the individual patient.

The eight components of comprehensive nursing care just introduced will be discussed in the succeeding chapters. Analysis of the components is basic to the development of understanding of the unity of nursing care. Again, the parts, as knowledge of the disease alone, are not enough. They must be restructured and synthesized to achieve individualized care for the long-term patient according to his unique needs.

REFERENCES

1. Perrott, G. St. J., Lucille M. Smith, Maryland Y. Pennell, Marion E. Altenderfer, *Care of the Long-Term Patient*: *Source Book on Size and Characteristics of the Problem*. Washington, D.C.: Government Printing Office, PHS Publication No. 344. 1954. p. 7.
2. Fritz, Edna L., *Toward Better Nursing Care of Patients with Long-Term Illness*. New York: Division of Nursing Education, National League for Nursing. 1956. p. 23.
3. National Conference on Chronic Disease: Preventive Aspects, Chicago, 1951. *Conference Proceedings, Preventive Aspects of Chronic Disease*. Baltimore: Commission on Chronic Illness. 1952. p. 10.
4. Barker, Roger G., and Beatrice A. Wright, The Social Psychology of Adjustment to Physical Disability. *Psychological Aspects of Physical Disability*. James F. Garrett, ed. Washington, D.C.: Government Printing Office, Rehabilitation Service Series No. 210. 1955. pp. 18-32.
5. National Conference on Chronic Disease: Preventive Aspects, *op. cit.* p. 14.
6. Symposium on Theory Development in Nursing, *Nursing Research. 17*, 1968. pp. 196-227.
7. Ellis, Rosemary, Characteristics of Significant Theories. *Nursing Research. 17*, 1968. p. 218.
8. Beshers, James M., Models and Theory Construction. *American Sociological Review. 22*, 1957. pp. 32-38.
9. Ellis, *op. cit.*

2 OBSERVATION

Purposeful observation is one of the nurse's greatest assets and one of her biggest responsibilities. An essential part of the care of the long-term patient is to perceive, to recognize, to note, and to communicate facts and occurrences. Observation is basic to all other nursing skills. For instance, observation of the range of motion of the proximal interphalangeal joints of the hands of a patient with rheumatoid arthritis contributes to the plan of daily personal hygiene for the patient. Perception of the family relationships helps the nurse implement home care for a patient with multiple sclerosis. Observation of the physical arrangement in the kitchen of a mother with limited cardiac capacity assists the nurse in helping the patient achieve the prescribed reduction in the expenditure of energy.

Not only is observation an integral part of all nursing care; other people, too, depend upon the nurse's observations. The physician relies upon the nurse for determining the color of urine in the Benedict Qualitative Test in order to prescribe insulin dosage for the patient with diabetes. Nursing observations contribute to the physician's diagnosis of congestive heart failure. The social worker utilizes the nurse's perceptions of the family relationships when assisting a father with arrested tuberculosis to adjust to family life after hospitalization. The dietitian relies upon the nurse's observation of the anemic patient's eating habits in planning the patient's menu. Nursing observations are a basic part of the patient care given by all professional workers directly involved in the healing process.

Observation is the gathering of data for the purpose of identifying, clarifying, and verifying facts, events, and relationships pertinent to the care of the patient. It is a skill that the nurse must continue to develop if she is interested in the improvement of patient care.

Observational skills are developed through good basic instruction in the art of nursing and good supervision in the practice of nursing. (A good source of tools which can be used is Hildegard E. Peplau's *Interpersonal Relations in Nursing*.) Ultimately, the individual nurse is responsible for the quality of her observational skills and their use in nursing care.

The *sensitive nurse* is a term widely used. Many nurses are sensitive to patients on an intuitive level, but the skilled professional nurse—a good observer—is sensitive on a conscious level. She is able to perceive the needs of patients through the development and control of all of her senses.

Only a few people achieve more than a minimal development of their sensitivity. How many people have developed the sense of touch to the degree that the blind have? All of the senses—smell, hearing, vision, touch, sometimes taste, and the "sixth sense"—are exercised by the nurse in the process of gathering data about the patient. Through smelling a breath the nurse assists in the diagnosis of diabetic coma. Through hearing a patient's conversation with her husband, the nurse clarifies her impression of a marital relationship. Through tasting a prescribed salt substitute, the nurse deepens her understanding of the

OBSERVATION 17

patient's resistance to it and his continued use of regular salt. Through seeing changes in a patient's skin, the nurse receives warnings that help her prevent the development of a decubitus ulcer. Through the touch of a cold foot, the nurse discovers that rubber bands are being used for garters. Through her sixth sense a nurse can perceive many things—such as internal hemorrhage in a patient—although she has just walked into the ward.

Smell, hearing, vision, touch, and taste are well-defined senses; the "sixth sense" is not. A precise, widely accepted definition for this sense has not been formulated as yet, though the term is commonly used. Sometimes it is used as a synonym for intuition or extra-sensory perception. Some suggest that it describes the development of the five senses to a very high degree of sensitivity. An expression describing an unexplainable anticipation of impending disaster is, "There's something wrong, but I can't quite put my finger on it." This is the sensing of a charged atmosphere devoid of immediate, tangible, overt manifestations. Perhaps the sixth sense can be understood as the reception of one or more stimuli of which a person is consciously aware without being able to identify any of the stimuli or the process by which they were received or recognized. Some people have a highly developed sixth sense, while others have not. It is not known whether it is an inborn trait or one that can be developed. The lack of systematic, scientific data documenting the existence of the sixth sense precludes any definitive statement about it. However, this does not prevent the nurse from using it in her nursing care. No perception should be disregarded on the basis that the nurse cannot explain it. Every perception should be thoroughly investigated and validated or invalidated before judgment is passed or action taken.

Good observation depends not only upon the skill of the

nurse but also upon her being with the patient. The subtle changes in the patient's condition cannot be observed if the time spent with the patient is short, nor can marked changes be observed from the nurses' station. Although the nurse need not be with the patient every minute every day, the nurse-patient relationship does imply a closer contact than is common practice today. One reason for the indispensability of the nurse on the health team is the close, continual contact she has with the patient.

Contact with the patient is a relationship. Four types of relationships between an observer and the person being observed were first suggested by Lasswell. Peplau[1] applied them to nursing. The four relationships are:

(1) The *spectator* relationship is one in which the patient is not aware of being observed and the nurse is outside the patient's focus of attention; for example, a nurse may be attending to the needs of one patient in a ward and at the same time observing what another patient is doing without that patient knowing it and without the nurse's attitudes or behavior entering into the situation being studied. The nurse may be observing relations between two patients in a ward while taking care of a third patient and without the first two recognizing that they are under observation.

(2) The *interviewer* relationship is frequently used by nurses in clinics, in homes, when admitting patients to a hospital, and the like. The patient is more or less aware that he is being studied in some degree, that the nurse is taking note of what he is saying in response to the situation or to questions that are asked of him. The nurse may use a prepared admission form for gathering data or she may permit the patient to take the lead in yielding data about himself and his feelings in the new situation; when the patient recognizes that he is being studied the relationship may be thought of as an interview, according to Lasswell.

(3) A supervisor or director of nursing service often makes use of a *collector* relationship; that is, they make use of records or reports prepared by nurses about patients in order to learn what has happened in a particular situation. Staff nurses and students make use of case history material gathered by internes, specialists, or other professional workers, including other nurses. Partial impressions about patients are gathered through using these data from other than personal observation.

(4) In *participant* relationships the nurse engages in ordinary activities connected with nursing a patient and at the same time observes the relationship between the patient and herself. The patient may refer to interest in various kinds of events, books, plays, songs, and thus give the observer cues that cannot be observed directly. The patient is aware that he is receiving nursing when he receives a bath, an enema, or a catheterization, but he is not aware that his responses to the procedure and to the attitudes of the nurse giving it are being observed directly.

The nurse caring for the long-term patient may utilize any of the four relationships mentioned here—the spectator-relationship, the interviewer-relationship, the collector-relationship, or the participant-relationship.

Observations made by the nurse must be organized into a general framework. Each observation must have a focus. Random observations (*e.g.*, what brand of clothing a patient wears) waste energy and serve no purpose. A system of observation facilitates the setting of time and place for each observation, insures a total picture of the patient, and gives meaning to each observation. One system of observation focuses on the patient as a special entity or on the patient in relation to others, in relation to the environment, or in relation to time. All four foci are important in the care of the long-term patient.

The patient observed as a special entity

Observations of the patient as a special entity are concerned with such items as the patient's reactions to drugs and treatments, the patient as a biological organism, or the patient as harboring a disease process. The quantity of literature devoted to toxic reactions to drugs and complications from treatments is overwhelming. To give just three examples:

1. Monoamine oxidase inhibiting drugs react with foods that contain amines such as cheese or yogurt to produce an acute hypertensive crisis.
2. Thiazide diuretic in combination with digitalis produces the same signs of toxicity that digitalis does.
3. Orinase given in combination with sulfonamide produces a hypoglycemic effect.

Compounding the difficulty is the introduction of many new drugs each year. Sometimes these drugs have been inadequately tested, or sufficient information about them is unavailable. Another major problem is the increasing use of multiple treatments and multiple drug therapy. In any of these situations the nurse has had to assume the responsibility for observing the patient's reactions to drugs and treatments. At times she has had to stop a drug when untoward effects occurred. Though the nurse cannot possibly know each new drug and treatment, she must learn as much as is available about each new drug before she administers it.

The patient is a biological organism. He breathes, sleeps, eats, and eliminates. The nurse should observe the daily activities of the patient. How frequently does the patient's chart read, "Ate well"? Yet how many patients, sick, away from home, and eating institutional cooking, do ever eat well? Eating well is very important to the therapy of the patient who has congestive heart failure, diabetes, or anemia. Minute, undramatic observations of activities of daily living greatly affect the long-term patient's condition.

Observations of the patient as an organism harboring a disease process are best known by most nurses. Observations which are diagnosis-oriented are the result of the disease-centered approach to patient care. They are essential as far as they go, but they are too limited and inadequate for comprehensive patient care. When observations are overly influenced by immediate diagnosis of the patient, equally important observations may be missed or overlooked. This is a critical omission in nursing care, particularly in view of the high incidence of multiple diseases characteristic of the long-term patient. Observations, regardless of diagnosis, should be all-inclusive.

The patient observed in relation to others

Even though the patient is in the hospital, relationships with others continue. These social relationships influence his condition for better or for worse, depending upon the situation. Perceiving, recognizing, and noting these relationships is a nursing responsibility. How does the patient react after visiting hours? Is he jovial? Is he sullen? Is he upset? Does a woman patient become more demanding of the nurse's time after her mother's visit? How many nurses utilize visiting hours for a view of the patient from the spectator-observer position? Family counselling greatly depends upon the nurse's observation of family relationships.

The relationships of the patient with the members of the health team comprise another important sphere.

The pregnant nurse who observes and identifies a strained relationship between herself and a woman patient who has had a stillborn child can help the patient in many ways. Observation of the patient will show in whom she confides her problems; this may indicate that the nurse is or is not fulfilling her responsibilities. Is the woman who scrubs the floors the one who listens to the patient because the nurse has too many other duties? The nurse can also help by smoothing out relationships between patients and doctors. In a teaching institution the patient may become upset by the visit of the teaching physician and five or so medical students. Yet the patient may accept teaching rounds if the nurse is aware of the patient's negative feelings and helps him work them through.

The patient in a hospital has relationships with many people: nurses' aides, dietitians, doctors, lab technicians, housekeeping personnel, and three shifts of nurses. The nurse must observe these relationships. She must also look for the effects of the patient's hospitalization on the relationships that the patient had before. There are four major possibilities: 1) A strengthening of a relationship (this may occur between husband and wife as a result of an injury suffered by the wife in a car accident). 2) A dependence upon a relationship by the patient or by the other person (a son may become more and more dependent upon his mother due to a diagnosis of multiple sclerosis). 3) A straining of a relationship (a wife may develop a strained relationship with her husband who has just had a colostomy). 4) A disintegration of a relationship (development of arthritis in a spinster may precipitate the disintegration of a previously strained relationship with her sister). Whatever the effect of a relationship upon a patient, the nurse has a duty to perceive it.

The patient observed in his environment

The third focus of observation is on the environment. This includes sound, air circulation, temperature, light, height of objects, safety of objects, and the distance between the patient and objects. These factors directly influence the nursing care of the long-term patient. For example, since room temperature and air circulation are essential in the care of the patient who has multiple sclerosis and who must be guarded against upper respiratory infections, the nurse must always be aware of these factors. Determining the correct height for the patient's bed aids the nurse in preventing falls and in promoting ambulation for the elderly patient who has had a cerebrovascular incident. Placing a television set within range of the patient's field of vision is important to the nurse's success in encouraging diversion for the patient who has congestive heart failure. A firm mattress helps the nurse maintain proper positioning for the patient who has rheumatoid arthritis.

An ideal environment is not always possible for the patient. A patient may require hospitalization and may also be needed at home. If a patient is on home care, a window looking out upon the street would help to divert him, but if he has a rear apartment, the nurse should not become discouraged. Within the reality situation, she should untiringly try to improve and control the patient's environment. To achieve this, keen nursing observations are essential.

The patient observed in relation to time

Time has different meanings to different people. If a patient arrives at the clinic five hours or a day late, obviously time has a different meaning for him than for the nurse. To such a patient, time may be vague and relatively unimportant. The nurse must consider this as a cultural difference. On the other hand, a patient may demand his medication exactly on time. Observation of this patient may disclose a rigid code of time and punctuality. In this situation the nurse should give the medication exactly when it is due. The detection of subtle physical, psychological and sociological changes in the long-term patient implies long periods of time, measured in weeks, months, or even years. For example, the arthritic involvement of an additional digital joint may occur over a period of six months. The disintegration of the relationship between a husband who has Parkinson's disease and his wife may take place over a period of years.

Communicating the observations

The communication of discriminating, accurate, and complete observations pertinent to the care of the patient is the final stage of the total concept of observations. Regardless of the quality of the observations, their relevance to the patient's care, and the conscientiousness of the nurse, observations are worthless unless they are communicated and integrated into the plan of the patient's care. Communications include the nurse's professional judgment in regard to the content to be conveyed, the appropriate people to contact, the time to report, and the method of reporting —in other words, "what," "to whom," "when," and "how." These four aspects of communication are determined by the nature of the observations, such as an emergency observation in the instance of a post-operative hemorrhage or a non-immediate but important observation in the case of the final healing of a decubitus ulcer.

OBSERVATION

The nurse must use keen professional judgment in deciding which observations are essential and which are not. It is common to read in a chart, "Mr. Jones in Room 320 was admitted at 5:30. Diagnosis: rheumatoid arthritis. Two aspirin at 7:00 for pain." The nature of the pain is not stated; neither is the site nor whether the pain was present upon admission or whether it is related or unrelated to his arthritis. A report on the effect of the aspirin and the duration of relief, if any, is lacking. No mention is made of other comfort measures which were tried nor of their effectiveness; for instance, we are not told what attempts at positioning were made. While reporting the pain is essential, the lack of substantive reported data makes the communication meaningless. A good guide for the content to be reported is the question, "What would I need to know if I were the next nurse responsible for the care of this patient?"

Communicating with the appropriate person can be simple or complex. Toxic reactions to drugs are reported to the doctor who ordered them. Communicating observations such as the patient's desire for a glass of warm milk before going to sleep lies in the nurse-to-nurse or nurse-to-ancillary realm. Some observations, such as a patient's capacity for, and attitude toward, learning new patterns of daily living are best communicated in the health team conferences. Others, such as a nurse's observation of a patient's need to work through her feelings about her altered body image following a radical mastectomy, may involve only one, or sometimes all, of the members of the health team. The roles played by different people on the health team vary from team to team and, within a given team, from patient to patient. See the chapter on counseling for a discussion of the health team.

In reporting observations of an emergency nature, the time element is clear and obvious. However, most of the observations made during the care of long-term patients are less immediate in nature and less obvious. Changes in the patient's condition are so subtle day-by-day that they seem unimportant or are overlooked completely. Observations of the long-term patient should be reviewed and summarized at regular intervals, and at shorter intervals after any critical periods, such as intermittent acute exacerbations. These summaries should be based upon the nurse's continually made and recorded observations. The specific time periods between reviewing periods vary from agency to agency and from institution to institution; they should be determined by the patient's illness, type of therapeutic regime, and individual needs.

There are two basic methods of communication: the oral form and the written form. Both methods range from very informal to very formal in structure and format. Both demand succinctness, accuracy, intelligibility, and thoughtfulness. Oral communications take such forms as telephone calls, patient conferences, and face-to-face encounters. Written communications include interagency referrals, follow-up reports, progress reports, and patients' records.

The importance of the patient's written record cannot be stressed enough. Most nurses react to the word "recording" with the comment, "Oh, no! Not that! Nobody reads the patient's record, anyway." True, records are often not read; but this is usually because they contain no significant observations or data. The record that reads "no complaints" conveys more about the nurse who wrote it than about the patient. The patient's record should compensate for the frailty of the human memory: it is an impossibility for any nurse to remember without a written record all of the pertinent data about a public health case load of fifty patients over a period of time—or even for ten patients for whom she is team leader for a day.

OBSERVATION

The skills requisite to writing good patient records are difficult to develop. Any meaningful writing requires time for thought, organization, expression, and legibility. This requires time which should be adequately provided for within the nurse's working hours. During the initial development of writing skills, which requires good supervision and periodic evaluation, it may take as long or longer to record the observations as actually to make them.

Observation of the long-term patient forms a basis for his care. Many nurses have highly developed observational skills but deny that this is so because they do not know what to do with them. The nurse does not always have the full responsibility for action that is indicated by her observation. Thus, treatment for toxic reactions to drugs is the doctor's responsibility, whereas accurate observation of the patient's reactions and communicating these to the doctor is the nurse's responsibility. The nurse must recognize these limitations of her professional responsibility—a responsibility which many times is restricted to perception, recognition, and communication of her observations to others. At other times the professional responsibility of the nurse includes direct independent action. Observation, the basic skill component in the nursing care of the long-term patient, flows from a close, continual contact with the patient—a contact which the nurse should cherish and protect.

REFERENCE

1. Peplau, Hildegard E., *Interpersonal Relations In Nursing*. New York: G. P. Putnam's Sons. pp. 273-274.

3 PHYSICAL CARE

What does the nurse do? Historically, the nurse began by employing her manual skills to alleviate the suffering of the sick. These skills were expanded later to include helping to prevent complications and to eliminate disease. Gradually the nurse's skills came to include the promotion of health and the prevention of disease. Currently, she does many things, though one image of the nurse has never been lost—"the laying on of the hands."

Physical care, "the laying on of hands," includes bodily care of the patient—bathing him, assisting him to the bathroom, helping him to feed himself. The nurse must be alert to the patient's normal bodily needs as well as to the special needs caused by a long-term illness, and she must be an expert in meeting both needs. For instance, for proper sleeping positions, the normal need is for a firm mattress, freedom of movement, and loose but sufficient bedding. The long-term patient who has had a cerebrovascular incident with a right-side paralysis needs the normal sleeping position *plus* a foot support to prevent foot drop, some apparatus to assist him in moving from side to side, and a special way to secure the bedding. The ways of meeting the patient's needs might include the installation of a foot board, a trapeze, a foot cradle, and pleating the top covers at the foot of the bed.

PHYSICAL CARE 29

Even though physical care tends to be relegated more and more to ancillary and nonprofessional personnel, it is still the ultimate responsibility of the professional nurse. It may be the most crucial and challenging aspect of the patient's care, requiring an alert mind, a flexible spirit, and much ingenuity. The long-term patient, by the nature of his disabilities and the length of nursing time required, presents a challenge to the professional nurse. For instance, the care of the hair requires daily attention and contributes to a person's self-esteem. However, the patient who has rheumatoid arthritis may be unable to reach her hair for combing, washing, and setting. If it becomes matted, it is not only uncomfortable and damaging to her personal esteem, but also interferes with optimum recovery. The ultimate solution to this nursing problem may be through the use of self-help devices or the services of relatives, friends, or beauticians. It may not be easy to find the solution, but to do so is essential to the welfare of the patient. Any nurse who has witnessed a patient's reaction to the solution of personal care problems knows how relieved the patient feels, how it contributes to his progress, and how rewarding the experience is for the nurse.

During the course of a long-term illness the patient is in intermittent contact with the nurse through periodic hospitalization, office or clinic visits, or services given by the nurse in the patient's home, but his personal needs are present hour by hour and day by day. Therefore, the nurse should aim for maximum independence on the part of the patient in caring for his own personal needs. In other words, the nurse should try to "work herself out of a job." Optimum self-care should be the ideal in each of the following categories of physical care: environmental control, bodily protection, feeding, toileting, bathing, exercising, and support and positioning.

1. *Environmental control.* Environmental control is a category of physical care that was defined and strongly advocated by Florence Nightingale. Temperature, ventilation, sounds, lighting, colors, furniture design, and proximity to other people influence the health of every person. The environment affects the long-term patient even more than the healthy person and is often more important. Though the nurse is neither an engineer nor an architect, she needs to be acquainted with basic environmental controls and must act upon this knowledge.

More and more, nurses are being consulted in planning hospital wards and nursing homes. The selection of the most desirable room for a patient in the hospital should be based upon the patient's condition. There is no rationale for leaving a patient in the room to which he was admitted. Transfer may appear to be burdensome, but, if indicated, the benefit derived by the patient will result in less time and effort spent by the staff and, ultimately, in a better prognosis for the patient.

Adaptations in the basic environment for a specific patient can be either the full responsibility of the nurse or one shared with other members of the health team. In either case the adaptations are dependent upon the patient's illness and his personal preferences and desires.[1] For example, if the patient has multiple sclerosis, control of the room temperature and air circulation is extremely important to prevent that most fatal complication, an upper respiratory infection. Or, for the patient who is going home after hospitalization for congestive heart failure, changing his bedroom from the second floor to a den on the first floor will not only facilitate the serving of meals but will provide the patient with some social involvement in and stimulation from the household activities. It will also eliminate the obstacle of stairs when ambulation is prescribed. When determining

PHYSICAL CARE

and implementing the patient's environmental needs, the nurse must take into consideration the patient's safety, his social requirements, his therapeutic needs (which are determined by his personality and illness), and the available facilities.

2. *Bodily protection.* Protection of the patient's body is achieved through draping, dress or clothing, and covering such as bedding. Specific techniques of draping, appropriate for physical examinations, treatments, and the like, are found in the literature. Whatever method of draping is employed, the nurse should give as much attention to the patient's comfort and modesty as to the method. For example, in preparing a patient for a vaginal examination, the upper part of her body should be warmly covered with a sheet or blanket which will stay in place while allowing freedom of movement. Some protection such as cotton bootees or paper slippers will provide comfort to her feet while in the foot supports. The draping of the legs should include some padding between the back of the patient's knees and the stirrups. The patient's modesty is respected by covering the perineum when she is not being examined. How familiar is the comment, "I was embarrassed to tears. Why, I must have been on that table, freezing, for half an hour, waiting for the doctor to see me."

Another area of protection is dress or clothing. The literature on rehabilitation contains much useful information about clothing designed for specific patients' needs. For instance, elastic shoestrings for the patient unable to reach his feet or to manipulate his fingers to tie the shoestrings are on the market at a reasonable cost. Many times the nurse will have no resource which provides the specific solution to the patient's problems in dressing himself. By exercising a little ingenuity, by seeking outside advice and resources, and by involving the patient in the solution of his particular needs, the nurse will find that the majority of the patient's dress and clothing problems can be solved.

The last area of protection is covering such as bedding. One of the first nursing arts that the nurse learns is how to make a bed. The long-term patient will require certain adaptations in bed-making, particularly if he is receiving treatments through tubing or catheters. The essential elements remain: a dry bottom sheet free from crumbs, wrinkles, and tears; loose, non-restrictive, though secure, top covers; adequate warmth. Meticulous attention to the bed of the patient not only contributes to his comfort but also promotes good skin care.

3. *Feeding.* Feeding comprises another category of physical care activities. Every individual has a set of attitudes toward food which were formed early in life and which he carries with him throughout his life. Some of these attitudes and beliefs were determined by cultural factors and others by emotional, religious, or other factors.

One woman may look upon the preparation of food as the activity that symbolizes her womanhood, her motherhood, her role in life. When deprived of this function she may feel she has lost one of the most important elements of her social role and her individual identity. Thus, when in a home for the aged she is allowed no access to or responsibility for the kitchen and food, her role changes and she may express her distress in many ways, one of which may be open, angry criticism of the food served in the home. There are other examples. Some holidays are not really holidays unless certain foods (such as roast turkey on Thanksgiving) are prepared, served, and eaten. Some religions forbid certain foods—Jews and Moslems, for example, are not

PHYSICAL CARE

allowed to eat pork. Some patients dislike certain foods because they associate them with unpleasant childhood memories—orange juice with cod liver oil.

In addition to a set of attitudes and beliefs, each person also has a set of motor skills which allow him to feed himself. For most healthy individuals, eating is an effortless, pleasurable activity, but for the long-term patient eating can become a difficult problem, taking a long time and requiring thought and changes in attitude. The nurse may have to tube-feed or hand-feed the patient, or help him to feed himself. A good reference for the nursing responsibilities for tube feeding can be found in *Medical-Surgical Nursing* by Shafer, Sawyer, McCluskey and Beck.[2] In feeding the patient, the nurse must be gentle, thoughtful in offering food according to the preference of the patient, understanding of the patient's likes and dislikes, and unhurried.

The ideal goal in feeding the patient is that he should assume total responsibility for feeding himself. For this he may have to learn new patterns of muscular coordination. He may require self-help devices such as a built-up knife, fork, and spoon. He will need patience, encouragement, and praise from the nurse. At times the nurse will need to restrain herself from helping the patient in order to promote his developing independence. Rather than feed the patient herself, though it may be efficient at the time, the nurse should verbally encourage him as he struggles to put a piece of meat on a spoon and struggles again to get the spoon from the plate to his mouth.

Attitudes towards food, realization of role changes, mechanical difficulties, physical impairments—all may impede the patient's dietary regime. The nurse must be alert to these therapy-blocking factors and find a way to ease or eliminate them.

4. *Toileting.* Toileting activities constitute another category of physical care. Regular and adequate elimination is frequently disrupted during the course of a long-term illness. Constipation may be caused by a decrease in physical activity. Diarrhea may be caused by a change in the diet. Excessive urination may be caused by medication. The first nursing activity is to provide the patient with the opportunity to void or have a bowel movement. The importance of this is illustrated by the experience in a large urban rehabilitation hospital where a research study was conducted to determine the need for a bowel and bladder rehabilitation program. In response to the question, "Are you incontinent?" every patient on one ward replied, "Yes." But before the bladder retraining program was started, the nurses' aides decided to offer the patients bedpans every two hours. After that action, not one patient was "incontinent," and the bowel and bladder rehabilitation program was never instituted.

If the patient is on absolute bedrest, the bedpan should be offered to him at frequent regular intervals. Except in illnesses which require very restricted activity and specific bodily positions, such as the acute phase of shock after a myocardial infarction, a commode is preferred. More energy is expended in getting on a bedpan than in sitting on a commode. Portable commodes are very useful; a bedpan placed on a chair beside the bed will serve the same purpose if safety precautions are observed.[3]

Assistance to the toilet is another activity. The nurse should consider the distance from the patient's bed to the toilet. For example, in assisting the family at home to prepare for the care of the father who has had a cardiovascular renal disease, the major factor in the selection of his room should be its proximity to the bathroom. When all ways to promote natural elimination fail, other possi-

PHYSICAL CARE 35

bilities will have to be tried. Yet catheters, enemas, and medications should be a last resort and used only when there is no other way. The nurse should be familiar with bowel and bladder rehabilitation. Many patients are now deprived of such rehabilitation because nurses lack knowledge and training in it. Toileting activities must never be overlooked. The human body is too intricately balanced to allow inadequate elimination patterns to develop and thereby further complicate the patient's condition.

5. *Bathing.* Another category of physical care is bathing; this includes the care of the skin, hair, nails, mouth, eyes, and nose. The daily bath is a phenomenon of our culture. The advocates of the daily bath will say that people are "refreshed" after the bath. But not everyone is. As regards bathing, some patients are more aware of the nurse's needs than she is of theirs. A classical comment from a patient in response to a nurse's questioning about the bath is, "Are you going to be like my last nurse? She always felt so much better after I'd had a bath." The frequency of the bath should be determined not only by the age of the patient but by his past bathing habits, his illness (whether frequent bathing is necessary or advisable), and by his wishes in the matter. In addition to the actual bath, attention should be given to the safety of bathing equipment such as hand rails on the tub, rubber matting on the floor of a shower, the type of soap, the temperature of the water, and the height of the tub or shower.

The patient's hair should be combed daily and washed frequently. Short hair or braids lessen the likelihood of matting and tangles. Care of a man's beard should not be overlooked.

The patient's nails should be trimmed and kept clean. Toenails present a big problem to elderly people and to patients who are unable to reach their feet or control their finger coordination. The patient should be referred to a chiropodist when the nails require more than normal care.

Maintenance of good oral hygiene is important. Glycerine and lemon juice is still a good cleanser. Opportunity for tooth brushing should always be provided for the patient restricted to bed, whether in a institution or at home. Consideration should be given to the condition of the teeth or dentures for they directly influence eating habits and food intake.

Bathing activities for the healthy, normal individual are relatively simple and taken for granted; for the patient with a long-term illness they become more difficult to accomplish and more important for the prevention of complications.

6. *Exercising.* The activities of exercising begin with the normal range of motion required by all average, healthy persons and extend to include complex exercises prescribed for a specific patient. Nursing responsibilities vary according to available facilities within the work setting. The nurse's responsibilities are, first, to initiate simple exercises based upon the doctor's appraisal of the patient's capacity for activity, second, to initiate specific exercises prescribed by the doctor and, third, to assist the patient in following a specific regime designed by the physiotherapist. During the bath most patients can easily tolerate the full range of motion; a series of activities will maintain muscle tone, stimulate bodily functions, and prevent muscular deformities. It will also promote good mental health.

A good source for range of motion exercises is the pamphlet *Strike Back at Arthritis.*[4] An example of specific exercises which the nurse can initiate upon prescription

PHYSICAL CARE

by the doctor are those designed to restore normal use of the affected arm of a patient who has had a radical mastectomy. These exercises are well described in the pamphlet *Help Yourself to Recovery*.[5] An example of a specific regime in which the nurse assists the patient is a series of shoulder exercises, designed and supervised by the physiotherapist, for the patient who is preparing to operate an artificial hand.

The nurse should be alert to the patient's exercise needs. She should know the basic elements of common exercises and understand the principles of specifically designed exercises. She needs to work with others to protect the patient from unnecessary loss of movement and insure the patient's maximum muscular control.

7. *Support and positioning.* The activities of support and positioning are focused upon both affected and non-affected parts of the patient's body. The goal is to promote the maximum amount of coordination and movement of the patient's body. The emphasis of nursing care should be placed upon maintaining the function of any part of the patient's body, whether it be an arthritic hand or a good foot and leg. In the care of an arthritic hand, a simple measure to prevent progressive contracture is to place a roll in the palm of the hand in a functional position. A classical example of caring for a good leg and foot is to insure maintenance of movement and strength through use of a commercial foot board or improvised equipment such as a slab of wood, a foot stool, or a box.

Nursing measures extend from the patient in bed to the patient who is beginning to ambulate. The transition from bed to ambulation is not easy for the patient. Fear is a big block to getting out of bed—fear of falling, fear of pain, fear of the unknown. Fear can be dispelled through motivation, through the patient's knowledge and understanding of equipment and the rationale behind it, and through successful experiences. Motivation is complex and depends upon variables such as the patient's background, preferences, and current living condition. The patient may refuse to give himself a bath because he wants the attention of his wife—attention offered only during the bath. (In the care of patients who had cerebralvascular incidents, Howard Rusk and his workers found that the strongest motivation for rehabilitation was the statement, "We can help you regain control over your bladder and bowels.") Instruction in the use of crutches and in the gait that the patient will use will help him become comfortable and skilled in their use. Understanding the reason for selecting the gait will reinforce an understanding of his particular diagnosis. A successful trip to the bathroom, accompanied by ease in getting out of bed and back, will encourage the patient to make repeated efforts to continue voiding in the toilet.

As an example of how these three phases can be combined into the care of an individual patient, consider the patient who asks about the birds singing outside his window. He might be motivated to get to the window to see them. If he knows which foot to put on the bed stool first, what the nurse will do to help him when he gets out of bed, and where to put his weight once he's on his feet, and if he realizes the necessity for increased circulation, he is provided with the essential facts and their rationale. Once he has been to the window, identified the birds, and returned to bed safely, he will feel the satisfaction that comes from a successful experience and his confidence in future ambulation will be strengthened.

Excellent physical care of the long-term patient is often deterred because the nurse sees little "glamor" in such activities. This view may be due more to a lack of immediate successful experience or of know-how on the part of the nurse than to the reality of the situation. Excellent physical care promotes the personal comfort of the patient and prevents complications, further injury, and deformities of unaffected parts of his body. It is sometimes difficult for the nurse to practice self-restraint as she helps the patient to help himself. The long-term patient may need to accept physical discomfort day after day due to the nature of his illness, but he should never have to do so because of a lack of nursing care. Physical care is important not only as one major component of nursing care but also as a basis for other nursing activities. The nurse must retain her one-to-one contact with the patient through physical care.

REFERENCES

1. Harmer, Bertha, and Virginia Henderson, *Textbook of the Principles and Practice of Nursing.* New York: The Macmillan Company. 1960. pp. 109-162.
2. Shafer, Kathleen Newton, Janet R. Sawyer, Audrey M. McCluskey, and Edna Lifgren Beck, *Medical-Surgical Nursing.* St. Louis: The C. V. Mosby Company, 1967. pp. 107-108.
3. Asher, Richard A. J., The Dangers of Going to Bed. *British Medical Journal.* Dec. 13, 1947. p. 967. Reprinted in *California's Health*, Oct. 15, 1958.
4. *Strike Back at Arthritis.* Washington, D. C.: Government Printing Office, PHS Publication No. 747. 1960.
5. Bernhardt, Ella, Terese Lasser, and Helen B. Radler, *Help Yourself to Recovery.* American Cancer Society. 1957.

4 EMOTIONAL SUPPORT

Emotional support is a term frequently used when nurses talk about patient care. Most nurses agree that emotional support for patients is important, and that everyone on the health team should provide it. Although the term "emotional support" is much used, its meaning often is not clear. However, if it is present, it can be easily recognized. It takes many forms: the interested question of the nurse who waits for the halting answer of the patient; her soothing hum as she cuddles the baby during feeding; her quieting hand on the patient's shoulder during a painful treatment or examination; her friendly greeting of the patient as he is admitted to the ward.

"Emotional support is not some sort of nebulous counseling; rather it is *action* directed at demonstrating interest, concern and respect."[1] The action may include two forms of communication, verbal and nonverbal. Touch has a language of its own. The "laying on of hands" has been known to be comforting for thousands of years. There is no reason to believe its effectiveness is any less in the 1970's. For example, a night nurse on a surgical ward makes rounds every hour. If a patient moves, she gives him a brief pat or touch. With others, she touches a foot as she passes the bed. When a catheter needs to be irrigated to release

EMOTIONAL SUPPORT   **41**

clots, this is quietly done; and as she leaves the bedside she gives a parting touch. No words are spoken, so as not to arouse the patients too much. When the patients recover, they frequently mention how comforting it was to know someone was around and checking on them.

As a part of sensitivity training at Esalen in California, touch for communication purposes is used as if it were a new discovery. Yet nurses have used this form of communication for decades.

At a conference on Nursing and the Liberal Arts sponsored by the New England Council on Higher Education for Nursing, contributions were made to nursing from the field of dance—in understanding what is said by the body without the use of words. The conscious use of touch to comfort is important. However, we need to read what body stance and position mean if we are to understand our patients.

Every little movement has a meaning all its own.
Every thought and feeling by some posture may be shown.[2]

Body language is a primary mode of communication. A person with a low evaluation of his worth may hang his head, avoid eye contact, hollow his chest, and slump his shoulders. Body language usually occurs together with verbal communication. It may express the same meaning as the spoken word or the opposite. An example of the opposite: the person moves forward, extends his hand, and then smiles without eye involvement. When the welcome is sincere, the smile occurs first, the chest rises, and then the hand is extended.[3]

Body language communicates powerfully. We can use it effectively, as in the following instance: "When she had crying jags, I would put my arms around her and hold her.

This seemed to help her gain control, and she would end by saying something like, "There I go again, bawling like a baby."[4]

When words are of little help, emotional support can be provided by the nurse's simply being with the patient. Though the nurse is not talking or doing anything, her presence alone can comfort the patient. Presence alone is not a simple thing. It brings with it a complex of non-verbal communication that can be very active, flowing from both the patient and the nurse.[5] By her body stance, the nurse can tell the patient she understands. The patient can tell the nurse he is frightened by the expression around his eyes or the wringing of his hands.

The nurse can learn much about the patient if she is sensitive to nonverbal areas of communication. Nonverbal communication may also set up blocks; for example, a nurse may already have one foot out of the door while the patient is struggling to tell her something.

It is important to learn to tolerate silence. Our noisy environment is not conducive to calm and quiet. Our ability to be quiet and calm is dependent on our own orientation. "No nurse can help the patient achieve inner growth, despite physical decline, unless she herself has some basic and sound concept of life."[6] The nurse needs to be quiet long enough to let the patient make his statement. When the patient has said only a few words, we rush in to answer what we think he is saying rather than what he is actually saying. Listening is a skill that can be taught and developed. Listening is the basis for clear verbal communication.

As teachers of nursing, the authors have had considerable experience in noting the developmental phases in listening and in verbal communication. We find that there are two types of occurrences as the student begins to interact with the patient. In one, the student gives a direct answer to

EMOTIONAL SUPPORT

a direct question, but without any awareness of the emotional overtones in the question. In the second, the student and patient talk on unrelated parallel lines without any touching of ideas. An example:

"Mrs. Kerr, I am going to change your dressing."
"Oh, Miss Campbell, I didn't sleep a wink last night."
"Will you please turn over on your right side?"
"I wonder what Charlie is doing today: he has trouble fixing his meals."
"There is less drainage on the dressing this morning."
"You know, he is such a baby with housework."
"Your stitches will come out tomorrow; that should make you feel good."
"I don't know what I am going to do when I get home. It will be quite a while before I can climb the stairs."
"There, this smaller dressing should make you more comfortable."

etc. etc.

The burden of the above interaction rested on the nurse. Obviously, the patient had some major concerns, but they were not heard. The nurse was trying to be reassuring, but the patient was unable to listen. Such an interaction is of little help to the patient, and probably is not very satisfying to the nurse, particularly when she becomes aware of the missed opportunity to be supportive. The patient was anxious. Anxiety can be displaced by the expenditure of physical energy, but this defense is not available to an immobilized patient. Since candor tends to dispel anxiety,[7] an honest, realistic open channel of communication between the nurse and patient might well have reduced the patient's anxiety.

There are times in patient care where listening with

sympathy should be the major activity. "It was not physical help this mother of five children, three of whom had muscular dystrophy, needed, but rather someone to talk with as one human being to another."[8]

The nurse need not be a psychiatric specialist to provide meaningful emotional support or to experience the satisfaction that comes from using herself therapeutically.[9] The ability to give emotional support to the long-term patient is dependent upon two factors. First, the nurse must have self-awareness, and second, she must be aware of, understand, and accept the wide range of reactions that are possible and likely in long-term illness. Each of these factors are complex and will be discussed in turn.

The self is used in all nurse-patient relationships. The self can be used in different ways. Some of the ways are detrimental to the patient; some are therapeutic.

What is therapy? It is the use of a means, such as a medication or a treatment, to heal the patient. Therapy cannot result from the use of the wrong tool or from an inappropriately used tool. The nurse must ask herself: "How therapeutically do I use myself? Do I use it like a precision instrument or a soothing ointment, or is it like a bludgeon or corrosive paste?" The more she knows about herself, the more she may use this self-knowledge in the patient-care situation and as a guide for her professional growth. For example, if a nurse knows the crying of children upsets her, then she should not seek employment in a pediatrics unit or in a nursery school. If she has emotional problems, she should not seek employment in a psychiatric hospital, thinking she may receive help there. Remember, the nurse is in nursing primarily to serve the patient and his needs. If the nurse needs psychiatric help, she should seek this help directly, and not indirectly through the ill patient.

Understanding oneself is never easy and is a life-long process. There are tools available to help the nurse in the growth of self-knowledge. Analysis is one of them; it is useful but not an end in itself. Analysis must be followed by synthesis and then by change of behavior. If the nurse is pulled apart by analysis and left in pieces, no benefit occurs either to the nurse or to the patient. However, analysis is a necessary first step to the understanding of the self. Help can be obtained from the self-analysis tools developed in the areas of human relations, small group behavior, industrial management, and psychology. Maslow's hierarchy of needs is well known and is frequently taught in classes.[10] But the question is whether the nurse who is able academically to list these needs is aware of her own needs. (Could you be specific if a close friend asked you to list your needs?) Awareness of needs is vital if one is to have control of how those needs are met. Think of the nurse who has a dependency need, as many do, and must give-give-give to her patients to keep them close even though they should be pushed toward independence for their own rehabilitation needs.

The nurse must ask herself, for purposes of analysis, how necessary it is to see progress in the patient's condition as a reward for the care she has given or to prove that she is a "good nurse." The nurse should know if it is necessary for her to be thanked or respected by the patient. Are the satisfactions from her personal life so meager that the nurse must demand affection from the patient? In what ways does the nurse allow the patient to express his gratitude?

We have observed that some nurses frequently receive gifts from their patients while other nurses who have developed equally close and helpful relationships with patients only rarely receive gifts. Apparently some nurses are unable to accept verbal thanks when offered or to communicate to the patient that their satisfactions lie in matters other than gifts. The issue discussed here is not that a professional responsibility exists in relation to gifts from patients but that the nurse's own needs determine her actions with the patients. Awareness of those needs will help her prevent confusion in the nurse-patient relationship and will keep her activities therapeutic for the patient.

Needs are closely intertwined with feelings. How does the nurse feel about the long-term patient? Is he a challenge or not? Many nurses do not realize that the incurable patient elicits antagonism as well as compassion.[11] It is difficult for the nurse to acknowledge that she feels revulsion or hostility when giving care to a mutilated patient. Such acknowledgment can be made and accepted and is the first step toward control or redirection of those feelings.

The care of Mr. Pelham is a case in point. He had cancer of the throat and lungs and a secondary pulmonary infection. His tracheotomy caused the evacuation of vast quantitites of foul smelling mucous. Because of his uncontrollable coughing, it was almost impossible to contain the mucous, which would spray the gown and bed. Two student nurses who were observing a demonstration of "trach care" with Mr. Pelham as the subject stayed during the entire procedure but were observed to turn pale. During a discussion of the incident at a post-conference session with their peers, they admitted their nausea and disgust. They were asked to think about how the patient producing the mucous and the spray felt. The students agreed that once they could speak about their feelings, they no longer felt so helpless about the situation. They recognized that the element of professionalism permitted them to act in spite of an initial revulsion, especially after the instructor admitted that she too felt like "gagging." The next day Mr. Pelham was given complete care by one of the students. The following day the student devised a way of folding a face towel around the tracheotomy so that there was less spraying and the mucous was more contained. The appearance and attitude of Mr. Pelham perceptibly improved, too.

The nurse's needs and feelings guide her actions and reactions. Many nurses wish to avoid long-term patients altogether. Or they may feel like neglecting them in favor of the other patients on the hospital ward or in the case load of the health agency. Another reaction is to overcompensate for the revulsion felt by being overly sweet to long-term patients—and perhaps developing a gastric ulcer in repressing that revulsion.

Death is a common occurrence in hospital wards with long-term patients. What does the nurse feel when she cares for the dying patient? How she views death determines the interaction with the patient and the quality of care. Yet, few nurses have stopped to answer the question of the meaning of death for themselves, and rarely do nurses try to see what death means for the patient and his family.

A nurse should make her self-knowledge available to the nursing service administration, and the information should be used in making assignments. For example, if a close relative of a nurse has just died, care of a dying patient should not be assigned to that nurse without talking it over with her. Similarly, the ability of a nurse to relinquish an assignment and request another when she sees she can no longer work with a particular patient is a sign of self-knowledge and the desire to maintain a therapeutic environment for the patient. Too often the request for a change is viewed as a sign of weakness. Nurses should follow in their profession the same principles of encouraging adaptations to change that they apply to patients.

The nurse must develop more insight about the negative and positive elements of judgment. She arrives at judgments from her observations and knowledge, and then she acts. She must not limit the knowledge to her personal feelings. She must be willing to change, to accept new evidence, and reorganize her picture of the patient and his needs. She may, for instance, decide on admission that a patient is not good material for rehabilitation, and refuse to admit later that she was wrong.

Knowledge of one's own personal judgment must be differentiated from the judgment one makes professionally. Awareness of personal judgments is the beginning of awareness of professional judgment. Personal judgment may have little therapeutic value to the patient. For example, if a nurse likes to keep her house clean, it does not follow that the patient should be made to keep his house clean. The professional judgment that a patient's house should be kept clean is made only insofar as it affects his health status. The nurse should be able to see, through the dirt, the health problem which needs solution and to use the positive aspects of the situation, e.g., the strong family ties, in her planning. If she lets the dirt interfere with the establishment of a working nurse-patient relationship, she may plan care based on her own needs rather than the needs of the patient.

Other examples of conflict between professional and personal judgment could be: the nurse who disagrees with Catholic philosophy and lets her feelings regarding birth control interfere with future teaching of the patient; or the personal view that all people from skid row are hopeless—so why try rehabilitation? "Why do I have to work with those dirty old men?"

The nurse's ignorance about the action (and reaction) of the self can be as dangerous to the patient as ignorance of the action of a drug. The addition of the self as a therapeutic tool in the nurse-patient relationship is a unique contribution the nurse can make to the care of the patient.

Besides developing an increasing knowledge of herself, the nurse must add another factor to her understanding if she is to care creatively for the long-term patient. The second factor is the ability to understand and accept the wide range of reactions that are possible and likely in long-term illness.

Fear is a large canopy under which the long-term patient exists. These fears have a stark reality. For example, there is nothing delusional about the fear that a colostomy is a deterrent to sexual intimacy.[12] Many women fear the mutilation of a mastectomy as much as they fear the carcinoma which makes the operation necessary. They fear that their husbands will no longer admire them after surgery.[13] Again, this is hardly delusional in a breast-conscious culture.

Any fear is real to the particular patient. As was stated, some fears are based on a specific change for the patient; some fears stem from old wives' tales which, to the patient, are a part of reality. All fears, expressed or hidden, are real, though some may be unfounded in fact. For example, a woman whose breast cancer is found early and eradicated may be so possessed by fear that she becomes an invalid.

When questioned informally and formally, patients list their fears usually in the following order:

1. pain and discomfort
2. the unknown
3. disturbance or destruction of body image
4. separation from normal environment
5. death
6. disruption of life plans
7. loss of control

8. finances[14]

Fear increases sensitivity to pain, and increased pain increases emotional excitement.[15] Direct intervention is necessary to break this recurring cycle. Since most fears stem from reality situations, false cheery assurances are of little value. The nurse who is sensitive in her observations, and evaluates how the patient really feels about his condition, can be of further help by giving the patient an opportunity to verbalize his feelings; this she would stifle by the reassurance that "everything will be all right." When patients are troubled, we alienate them if we divert their attention with a bright quip or a funny story. Such a light response tells the patient that his worries are trifling. We can make him feel alone in his suffering, surrounded by people who don't care, or we can try to understand him. A nurse who refuses to listen to a patient describe his feelings often does this from lack of understanding. Whether she rushes away, interrupts, or diverts the patient, she is not giving him the kind of support he needs. Human beings need someone to share with. The long-term patient has this need too. Through sharing, the misery is diluted. To be brave in an emergency is one thing; to be brave for years is different and more difficult. Some patients are required to be heroes every day.

The nurse may not be able to do anything specific to remove an expressed fear, but help is given when she lets the patient know she understands how he feels, and that she is interested in him. Listening to the patient express concerns and fears provide a safety valve for him. It also may provide information needed for planning treatment and further care.

Helplessness and dependency are experienced together by the patient. He feels helpless when he cannot care for his basic physical needs, such as feeding himself or going to the toilet alone. When he has severe pain, and perhaps strange tubes and gadgets coming from practically every body orifice, he is also completely dependent on the nurse. Dependency, if needed by a patient and denied him, is just as upsetting as the dependency position which a patient will not accept. It is important the patient be permitted to protest against the indignities to which he is exposed. Some patients, and we believe too many, are forced into keeping up a good front, being a "good patient," so the nurse will not reject them.[16] When a patient needs and demands attention, maybe he is the center of attention for the first time in his life. Let the nurse be aware of the need and supportive of the dependency, even if he is recovering beautifully.

Helplessness, loneliness, and boredom are common companions of the long-term patient. Denial and dependency are often present. Denial by the patient of the diagnosis or treatment offers him protection from overwhelming fear. The patient derives some protection from simple avoidance. For example, he will not look during the changing of the dressing after a radical neck dissection, to avoid seeing that he is no longer "whole." Or a woman may believe that rectal bleeding is not a sign of carcinoma of the rectum but a return of the menses. It must be emphasized that conscious denial does not necessarily reflect an unconscious awareness of the true state of affairs. An example of unconscious awareness is the patient with rectal bleeding who "knew from the beginning" that the bleeding was due to cancer.[17]

Other concerns frequently expressed by a long-term patient are about the future, what is happening to his self-image, and what implications the diagnosis has for his life in general and for treatment in particular. The future, the unknown, and the uncertain are more difficult for the patient to handle than the present.

As the patient discusses his concern for the future, his anxiety will lessen and he will be more able to accept and understand the nurse's explanation of hospital procedures, such as diagnostic tests, and the reasons for doing them.

When a patient loses a part of his body, the implications to him are profound. Each person has a body image which has developed over his lifetime, and which is closely tied to his feeling of self-respect. Any alteration in the body disturbs this image. A loss of a part of the body is viewed by the patient as a partial death. Depression is a frequent post-mutilation reaction—the patient is experiencing a period of mourning over the loss, the partial death. The loss may consist of a part of the body or of the function of a part of the body—either loss is important to the patient.

"Grief or mourning is a special kind of depression following a loss."[18] It is vital that the nurse not take steps to dissipate the depression but permit the patient to "do his grief work." The patient must be given time to express his sense of loss; only then can the pattern of adjustment occur. At first the patient will express such reactions as shock, denial, anger. These reactions should be expected and the patient should have the support and acceptance of the nurse. Crate has proposed that there is a model of adaptation to chronic illness and its resultant loss. The four stages are: 1) disbelief, 2) developing awareness, 3) reorganization, and 4) resolution and identity change.[19]

The identity change is often profound. With a change in the body image and a change in role it is easy to see the need for emotional support. An example may clarify the relationship between body image and role, which is the translation of status into behavior.[20] The father with a severe cardiac condition can no longer carry out the same activities. He may have to change his role from the employed to the unemployed, from the independent to the dependent, from the whole man to the incomplete man, and from the head of the household to a dependent. With a reduction of physical endurance, a change in the sex role can also be expected, with its resulting emotional overtones. Any change in the functioning of the body or in its completeness changes the patient's body image, an image that has been developing throughout his lifetime. With the image change, role also changes.

Two other factors also contribute to the emotional support of the patient, even though they are not often classified as such. They are 1) practice of the social amenities, and 2) spiritual support.

The social amenities are important. On admission to the ward, the patient can be relieved of some of his anxiety by a friendly greeting. Yet it is not uncommon that he overhears the admitting nurse make a remark like, "Oh, not another one!" Introduction to the other patients in the ward or room helps the new patient ease into a situation that carries many threats. As the period of hospitalization extends, the nurse must remember to acknowledge the presence of the patient when she enters the room, and not ignore him like a fixture on the wall. The nurse should call him by name when she passes the medications, and ask him to turn over for the injection rather than grunt at him.

Spiritual support, though it is not specifically emotional support, should also be mentioned. That part of the life which is called the soul or spirit, and matters of belief, hope, faith, and eternity, all have meaning to patients. Some patients need less spiritual support than others, but the nurse who ignores these areas does so to the detriment of the patient. Whether the nurse is able to give spiritual support is largely dependent upon her own spiritual condition. If the nurse does not feel comfortable in dealing directly with the patient's spiritual concerns, she must see that contact is made with an appropriate counselor. The nurse can do much to contribute to the physical and emotional setting for the observance of religious practices. Routines are useful but never enough. For example, the nurse may routinely call the priest for the Catholic patient who is dying, but overlook the fact that patients with other religious affiliations may also desire the presence of their minister or rabbi. Also, the patient who lists "no preference" or "none" for religion on his admission sheet may still need and want spiritual support.

Emotional support is directed at a constellation of highly charged beliefs, needs, fears, and reactions; more simply, emotional support is compassion in action.

REFERENCES

1. Field, William E. Jr., et al., The Senses Taker, *American Journal of Nursing.* 66:12, Dec. 1966. pp. 2654-2656.
2. Shawn, Ted, *Every Little Movement.* Pittsfield, Mass.: Eagle Printing and Binding Co. 1954. p. 10.
3. Christoggers, Carol Ann, Movigenic Nursing, An Expanded Dimension, in *Humanities and the Arts as a Basis for Nursing: Implications for Newer Dimensions in Generic Nursing Education.* New England Council on Higher Education for Nursing. June 1968. pp. 85-97.
4. Burnside, Irene Mortenson, The Patient I Didn't Want. *American Journal of Nursing.* 68:8, Aug. 1968. pp. 1666-1669.

5. Ruesch, Jurgen, and Weldon Kees, *Non-Verbal Communication.* Berkeley: University of California Press. 1956. 205 pp.
6. Fox, Jean E., Reflections on Cancer Nursing, *American Journal of Nursing. 66*:6, June 1966. pp. 1317-1319.
7. Davis, Robert W., Psychologic Aspects of Geriatric Nursing, *American Journal of Nursing. 68*:4, April 1968. pp. 802-804.
8. Kjos, Karen, Listening with Sympathy, *American Journal of Nursing. 66*:11, Nov. 1966. pp. 2471-2473.
9. Ujhely, Gertrude B., What is Realistic Emotional Support?, *American Journal of Nursing. 68*:4, April 1968. pp. 758-762.
10. Maslow, Abraham Harold, *Motivation and Personality.* New York: Harper Brothers. 1954. 411 pp.
11. Meyer, Bernard C., Some Psychiatric Aspects of Surgical Practice, *Psychosomatic Medicine. 20*, May-June 1958. pp. 203-214.
12. *Ibid.*
13. Barckley, Virginia, What Can I Say to the Cancer Patient? *Nursing Outlook. 6,* June 1958. pp. 316-318.
14. Carnevali, Doris L., Preoperative Anxiety, *American Journal of Nursing. 66*:7, July 1966. pp. 1536-1538.
15. Crowley, Dorothy M., *Pain and Its Alleviations.* UCLA School of Nursing. 1962. 80 pp.
16. Mauksch, Hans O., and Daisy L. Tagliacozzo, *The Patient's View of the Patient Role, Part I, Analysis of Interviews.* Dept. of Patient Care Research, Presbyterian-St. Luke's Hospital, Chicago. 1962. 69 pp.
17. Meyer, *op. cit.* pp. 203-214.
18. Kalkman, Marion E., Recognizing Emotional Problems, *American Journal of Nursing. 68*:3, March 1968. pp. 536-539.
19. Crate, Marjorie A., Nursing Functions in Adaption to

Chronic Illness, *American Journal of Nursing. 65*:10, Oct. 1965. pp. 72-76.
20. Christopherson, Victor A., Role Modifications of the Disabled Male, *American Journal of Nursing. 68*:2, Feb. 1968. pp. 290-293.

5 TREATMENT

Treatment as a component of comprehensive nursing care goes beyond a "how to" body of specific techniques. Knowledge is a necessary addition. Treatment, in our frame of reference, is a combination of both skills and knowledge. Treatment as a component of comprehensive nursing is, again, more than the addition of skills and knowledge. The whole of treatment is greater than the sum of its parts.

Treatment includes all of the specific measures applied in an attempt to diagnose and cure the patient—diagnostic tests, surgery, drug and diet therapy, radiation, mechanical manipulation, and limitation of movement of parts or all of the body, as in bed rest. To this must be added a concern for the economic aspects of treatment. Here knowledge of the sequence of diagnostic tests is vital. If, for example, a barium enema is scheduled before an I.V. pylogram, days of hospitalization are wasted, diagnosis is delayed, and the cost of the extra time often amounts to hundreds of dollars.

Whatever the treatment for the patient, it is always prescribed by the physician. As the nurse's knowledge of physiology increases, so does her function. Typical of this would be the advances that have been made in the treatment of the stroke patient by the use of stimulation with reflex response resulting in improved muscle tone.[1] The nurse's responsibility usually begins when she receives the prescription or "order." There are instances, though, in which her responsibility begins earlier—when her report of her observations of the patient provides the physician with information he requires for his initiation of a prescription.

It is the mechanics of treatment that often become separated and are thought of as the totality of treatment. The mechanics or specific manipulative skills are an important part of nursing. The mechanics can and should be taught to the family, the aide, or the licensed practical nurse. But the mechanics are taught in relation to a specific instance for a specific patient.

The wife of a patient who has had a cerebrovascular incident can usually learn to administer, and in turn teach the patient, the exercises the physician prescribes to keep the affected limbs supple. She can observe the nurse demonstrating the exercises, repeat the demonstrations, and take home the pamphlet *Strike Back at Stroke*,[2] which sells for less than a dollar. The physician should have marked on the pamphlet the exercises to do and their frequency.

Knowledge of a specific treatment for a patient does not make an individual a nurse. It is the competence to teach the specific in the total milieu, as part of her ability to practice all nursing components, that makes a person a professional nurse.

The nurse must be aware that she can often learn from the patient, particularly from the long-term patient, who has lived with his diseases for a period of time. The patient with an ileostomy who is hospitalized for an acute exacerbation of rheumatoid arthritis can give the nurse specific directions for the care of the ileostomy. When the nurse listens and follows his suggestions, she also contributes to his emotional support. An example of learning from

TREATMENT

the patient (a woman who was a quadriplegic, respiratory-post-polio, in for a cholecystectomy) is related in the literature:

A simple, "Will you tell me about yourself and your respiratory equipment?" gained my confidence. Of all the life-saving equipment that helped me, the presence of another human being was the most essential. In this age of electronic computers and monitoring machines, the intellect and compassion of a nurse are still the best healing devices.[3]

An analysis of treatment for several of the diseases that contribute to long-term illness, such as tuberculosis, cancer, arthritis, and cardiovascular disease, may show that they have one thing in common—complexity. Although there are, of course, ground rules for treating specific diseases, the treatment for each case is determined on an individual basis. The presence of multiple diseases in one individual complicates the treatment pattern. This will be discussed in the chapter on complex correlations.

The nurse must know the therapeutic procedures, the dosages and administration of medications, and possess the technical skill for manipulation of equipment. The knowledge and skills needed differ with each disease, and with the theory held on the treatment of that disease. Treatments that are in fashion in one part of the country may not be used in another. Expanding medical research contributes further to the fluidity of the treatment pattern for the long-term patient.

The nurse's position in treatment is a very crucial one, for it is she who actually administers drugs and treatments to the patient. What is taught in the school of nursing one semester may be out of date in the work situation the next. Keeping up with current treatment, therefore, is more important than knowing facts which may already be dated.

The ability to comprehend fully written directions and explanations is essential for the accurate administration of current medications. Reading for the sake of quickly gaining information is a special skill that needs cultivation. A notebook can be useful for keeping current information on drugs and treatment.

The question is sometimes raised, "If treatments are changed so rapidly, why bother to learn the specifics today?" First, because the nurse must care for patients today. For current practice her best sources of information are the latest editions of nursing books that give the details of procedures and techniques. Second, her knowledge of today's treatment is a base on which she can build her knowledge of tomorrow's. The understanding of treatment is enhanced by an historical perspective. A treatment in vogue today may be out of fashion tomorrow, but the day after tomorrow it may be re-established. For example, the Mantoux test, originally used clinically, was later used as an epidemiological tool. It went out of fashion for a couple of decades, but in the 1960's its definitive quality in differential diagnosis was recognized. It has been replaced in the 1970's by the Tine test, which differs in dosage and reading.

Time has changed the mechanics of therapy, but the needs of patients remain the same, as do therapeutic goals. The nurse is no longer cautioned to tuck the oxygen tent tightly around the head of the bed, but is taught to fit the nasal canula into the nares of the patient. Since a canula presents a problem when the patient is a mouth breather, the procedure requires more creativity from the nurse if the oxygen therapy is to be accomplished.

Time has increased the number of techniques the nurse practices. More and more of the treatments that were once the responsibility of other members of the health team are now part of nursing. For example, the nurse now observes

TREATMENT

the cardioscope and applies the pacemaker to the patient following open heart surgery. In contrast, only a few years ago the taking of the patient's blood pressure was the responsibility of the physician, as it still is today in some countries.

The following caution is given, not to underestimate the importance of technical knowledge and skills, but to put them in the proper perspective.

If we aren't careful, gadgetry may replace common sense. . . . The nurse needs to know more and more about defibrillation, artificial respirators, pacemakers, monitors, cardioscopes, direct recorders, and many other machines. Yet she must not allow the use of this dramatic equipment to infringe upon her bedside judgment and intelligent care of the patient. . . . Familiarity with the symptoms of coronary heart disease—its symptoms and care of the patient—should take precedence over familiarity with procedures of open heart surgery which is used in less than 1% of the total heart cases seen by the floor nurse in today's average hospital . . . We must never forget that none of our new equipment should replace the human mind, and that none of the computers can replace the human thought that created them.[4]

The nurse must look forward to further progress in therapy and increased responsibility in carrying out treatments. To handle the flood of new scientific knowledge and the changing procedures, the nurse should be able to ask and answer the following questions:

What treatment is ordered?
How is it to be administered?
What is the usual dosage of the drug or the usual routine of the procedure?
What is the expected therapeutic response to the treatment?

Are there dangers and toxic reactions from such a treatment?

If so, what, specifically, are they?

Does the patient have a history of an allergic reaction to the treatment prescribed?

How does one handle the equipment?

The nurse must seek information when she receives an order for a medication she has not given previously or does not immediately recognize. She is legally responsible for her actions and must make certain the medication and dosage is therapeutic before administering it to the patient.

The nurse has several sources of information. The first is the physician who orders the treatment. The second source is the hospital formulary or, if the medication ordered is too new to be listed, the hospital pharmacy. (Hospital pharmacists are now taking a more active role in the health team. Moreover, nurses are recognizing the legal implications of assuming any responsibility for the dispensing and labeling of drugs. Prepackaging of drugs and/or 24-hour coverage of the pharmacy by a registered pharmacist are very helpful in this area. Also, hospital pharmacists have recently increased their activity in staff education, and as a group are recognizing their responsibility to share their knowledge with the nursing staff. Joint conferences between hospital pharmacists and state ANA's are becoming more common.) The third source of information is the brochure printed by the drug manufacturers that accompanies the medication. These brochures are more useful for their description of chemical composition and general therapeutic effects than for clear listings of the toxic reactions that can occur. The brochures generally contain a bibliography and information on the sample number of patients used in the studies cited.

TREATMENT

What and how much is ordered? Is the order within the usual (safe) range of dosage for the patient? These basic questions are asked and answered first. The nurse next has to know upon which system in the body the treatment is expected to act. (The coined name of the preparation usually does not give her a clear clue. For example, although ornade sounds like ornase, it is a decongestant.) The nurse can then draw on her knowledge of normal physiology to observe the patient for both the therapeutic and toxic response to the treatment.

When the nurse knows the usual range of dosage and route of administration, she has a framework in which she can test the current order for the specific patient.

The pediatric dosage of isoniazid will hardly be effective for the truck driver weighing 200 pounds. The daily dosage of isoniazid for the toxic adult with newly diagnosed far-advanced pulmonary tuberculosis is not appropriate as a maintenance dosage for the adult whose tuberculosis is inactive and who is ready for discharge from the hospital.

Many drugs have a variety of routes of administration. If a certain drug is ordered by mouth and the pharmacy sends the drug to the ward in the form for parenteral administration, the nurse must recognize that there could be quite a difference in speed of response by the patient and seek further instructions from the physician or the pharmacist. Also, there are some parenteral preparations with slow absorption, e.g., procane penicillin or the new pellets for birth control which may last 20 years. Similarly, the time factor must be considered when the patient has been receiving a drug intravenously, and then the order is changed to suppositories.

Frequently, patients cannot understand that the medication is the same when the administration is different. Some patients object strenuously when the route of administration is changed or when the color or shape of an oral medication is different from that first received. The longer the patient has been receiving a certain form of a medication the more difficult it is for him to accept a change in the route, form, or timing of that medication. Skillfully explaining to the patient the reason for such changes is (generally) a nursing responsibility.

What is the expected therapeutic response of the patient to the treatment? The nurse must know *what* follows the treatment and *when*. When her expectations are clear she has a basis for her observational skills and can be accurate in reporting the patient's responses. The physician depends upon clear reporting on the response to a treatment ordered by him. He needs this information to form his own clinical judgment and to determine the further course of treatment.

Could there be toxic symptoms? What are the dangers to the patient? Even a brief survey of the current medical literature will show an alarming array of toxic reactions to drugs and treatments now in use. They range from slight transient reactions to such major threats as psychosis and cardiac arrest.

The nurse should expect certain kinds of toxicity from certain treatments. She will find, for example, the following reactions to steroid therapy listed in the medical literature: severe headache, dizziness, anorexia, purpura, weakness, fatigue, Cushingoid facies, diabetes, weight loss, peptic ulcer, and vertebral fracture resulting from osteoporesis.

From the rauwolfia preparations such side effects as diarrhea, nasal stuffiness, drowsiness, and psychic depression have been reported.

For the patient with inoperable cancer who is treated by x-ray or cobalt therapy, the nurse must watch for nausea, vomiting, rectal burning, and mild tenesmus. A knowledge of physiology makes us aware that x-rays destroy

TREATMENT 65

rapidly growing cells, and that, as the cells of the gastrointestinal tract are replaced approximately every four days, we can expect G.I. upset after x-ray treatment.

Diuretic therapy is often life saving. However, the nurse must be alert to problems that can result, such as: 1) electrolyte and water imbalance, 2) derangements of glucose metabolism, 3) retention of uric acid, 4) decrease in renal function.[5]

The probability that a new drug may produce toxic effects is high. When the nurse is alert to this probability, the patient is more likely to be protected.[6]

Does the patient have a history of an allergic reaction to the treatment prescribed? Allergy is unique for a specific patient; it is an adverse reaction to preparations with little or no known toxicity. It is important that the nurse question the patient about all of his known allergies before even such a "tried and true remedy" as aspirin is administered. Even sensitivity to adhesive tape must be determined to prevent excoriation of the skin around a wound area.

How does the nurse learn to handle the newer types of equipment? Again, she must seek information and practice opportunities from a variety of sources. The central service of the hospital often has instruction manuals, printed by the manufacturer, describing the use of the equipment. (However, instruction manuals can be overwhelming, as was true in the case of a 20-page booklet on care of the ileostomy bag recently seen by a nurse and patient. The problem was solved by the visits of a Q. T. club member who gave practical advice and who visited the patient after discharge.) Knowledge of the principles of physics relating to movement of gases, liquids, and pressure differentials can be useful. The best way to learn is probably by observing another person who understands the use of the equipment.

If practice in the handling of an apparatus is needed,

e.g., in the operation of the valves for Intermittent Positive Pressure Breathing, it should be arranged away from the bedside of the patient. His confidence in the nurse is increased by her ease and skill in handling equipment.

Again, the technical skills must be seen in proper perspective. The professional nurse must be able to question and seek clarification to assure safety and therapy for the long-term patient. She must also be prepared to relate the specific procedure to the total treatment plan for the recovery or rehabilitation of the patient.

REFERENCES

1. Elizabeth, Sister Regina, Sensory Stimulation Techniques. *American Journal of Nursing. 66:* 2, Feb. 1966. pp. 281-286.
2. *Strike Back at Stroke.* Washington, D. C.: Government Printing Office, PHS Publication No. 596. 1958.
3. Jeffris, Jane, The Best Healing Device. *American Journal of Nursing. 64:* 9, Sept. 1964. pp. 74-77.
4. Rawlings, Maurice S., Heart Disease Today. *American Journal of Nursing. 66:* 2, Feb. 1966. pp. 303-307.
5. Schneider, William J., and Barbara A. Boyce, Complications of Diuretic Therapy. *American Journal of Nursing. 68:* 9, Sept. 1969. pp. 1903-1907.
6. Rodman, Merton M., The Rising Tide of Dangerous Drug Reactions. *Nursing Forum. 1,* Winter 1961-62. pp. 105-127.

6 TEACHING

To make the point that teaching is an essential function of nursing care may seem superfluous, but the importance of teaching for the long-term patient cannot be overstressed. Some recent comments from the nursing literature call the vital nature of this nursing function to mind: "Truly good nursing is teaching," says Mary Lou Moore,[1] and Frances J. Storlie says, "It seems to me that teaching and nursing are inseparable."[2] In her book, *The Teaching Function of the Nursing Practitioner*, Margaret Pohl notes that an essential part of practice is effective teaching.[3] Teaching is not only necessary; it must be *planned* teaching. In an article on teaching the patient about open heart surgery, Filomena Vavaro suggests "that teaching be planned and that it become an integral part of the patient's nursing care."[4] Prior to open heart surgery, she reports, there is a three-day schedule of teaching. The family is included, and audio-visual equipment is used. Teaching is important to the long-term patient because he will have to take an active part in his continued treatment. When an acute illness is cured, the period of convalescence rarely is long and extended rehabilitation seldom follows. However, in long-term illness, a protracted convalescence or period of retraining of muscles and an adjustment to activities of daily living can be expected. The nurse's teaching aims at making the patient a partner in his nursing care. The goal is to help the patient become well-informed and skilled in the management of his disease and the maintenance of his health. There are many specific details the long-term patient must know about his disease. The nurse has this knowledge or knows where to obtain the information. The long-term patient usually needs follow-up care. Here, the nurse can implement the planning of home care by her knowledge of community agencies.

All of these teaching needs of the patient with long-term illness will be developed further. Before we discuss such planned teaching activity, let us look at the unplanned teaching the nurse does in any nurse-patient interaction.

The nurse is constantly teaching by her actions, her replies to questions, her directions to the patient, and her manner of interaction. She may teach the patient that the medications the doctor ordered are of little value by shrugging her shoulders when the patient asks about the purpose of the drugs. She may imply to the patient or his family that the changing of the colostomy dressing is so distasteful that the patient would do everyone a favor by dying. Or that the paraffin packs for the crippled hands of the patient with severe rheumatoid arthritis are just too complicated and messy to try to continue them when he goes home. Or that the exercises done in the physiotherapy department are so complete that it is not necessary to continue exercising on the ward. She may also imply, by her stance as she leans forward to hear the halting reply of the patient, that she is interested and concerned. Her encouraging smile as the patient puts on his leg brace tells him that he has learned. Her questions, as she removes the lunch tray, reinforces the patient's interest in nutrition and diet.

TEACHING

The nurse must be aware that she continually teaches, and must learn to direct the teaching. Self-knowledge (discussed in the chapter on Emotional Support) is a valuable asset for the nurse. She has to be able to "see" her teaching activities. This applies to unplanned as well as planned teaching. Sometimes it seems miraculous that patients are able to do what nurses desire when all the teaching is in complex medical-technical words. A useful, simple method to help the nurse see how she teaches is process recording. All she needs is paper, pencil, time to write, and the desire to hear what is said. This is what she does: After a short interaction with a patient, the nurse writes down everything she and the patient said, and makes some indication of how it was said. (As she practices recording, her memory for exact words and tones will improve.) Then she reads her notes critically. Probably her response will be: "Did I say that?" or, "How could I have missed the meaning of that statement?" Of course, having the recording read and discussed by a friend or teacher will speed up the analysis of the interaction. For a complete treatment of the process of listening and recording, see Peplau[5] and Rogers.[6]

The nurse is interested in having the patient change his behavior as a result of her teaching and his learning. Understanding an idea or fact does not necessarily bring about a change of behavior. How frequently we see the patient who *knows* what his diet should contain and repeats the instructions correctly but makes no change in his eating habits! Awareness of this phenomenon should not discourage the nurse from teaching but should help her face the reality that to achieve behavior change is the most difficult part of the teaching-learning process.

The teaching-learning process is built upon principles (learning-motivation, objectives-methods) that are readily available in basic textbooks on psychology and teaching. The practitioner is urged to review this material periodically to reinforce her own learning and to increase her effectiveness in patient teaching.

There are a few simple guidelines the nurse can use to improve her planned teaching. These consist of an adaptation of a formal teaching plan used by teachers in a school setting. The four headings are:

Content	Method	Materials	Questions

Content includes the *what*, the knowledge or skill (the substance) to be taught. *Method* includes the *how*, the way the content is to be presented—by demonstration, lecture, role playing, or other means. *Materials* includes the *stuff*, the equipment used to implement the method, e.g., pamphlets, models, motion pictures, or recordings. *Questions* is a guide on what to ask the patients during the teaching process in order to reinforce learning or to evaluate teaching.

If the nurse keeps in mind the four-column plan, she will not skip the vital steps in method and materials that help communicate the content.

As the nurse begins to plan her teaching she listens to the patient. She "listens" with her entire body and mind. The facial expression and body positions of the patient must be seen. The difference in tone in which certain words are spoken by the patient must be heard. The emotion expressed by the patient must be felt. The meaning of the questions the patient asks must be understood by the nurse's receptive mind. Listening can be learned and made increasingly useful in the nurse-patient interaction. A particularly valuable aid to the development of this skill can be found in *Listening with the Third Ear*, by Theodor Reik.[7]

As the nurse listens, she asks questions to clarify what the patient said; and again she listens. She does this with the purpose of learning exactly how much the patient already does or does not *know* about a specific idea or fact. Before the nurse demonstrates a skill necessary for the patient to learn, she questions and listens. She asks the patient for a demonstration and observes him. She observes and listens with the purpose of learning exactly what the patient *can do*. Only when the nurse knows explicitly what the patient knows and can do has she reached the beginning point for her teaching. Avoidance of this exploratory phase will often result in the nurse's talking over the patient's head or boring him with something he already knows.

By listening and observing, the nurse learns *what* the patient knows. She also comes to some conclusion about the length of his attention span and about his facility with words.

The kind of words the patient uses determines the form in which to present the teaching content, the *what*. But the nurse should not assume that a highly educated patient necessarily understands the basic principles of health, nor that an uneducated man may not already know and practice these principles. Listening and questioning is necessary, whatever the level of the patient's education. Avoidance of all technical or complex terms is not necessary—any unknown term may be used if it is explained in words the patient understands.

The same explanation or demonstration will not be successful with every patient. One cannot teach by rattling off a neat explanation. The nurse must know what she is trying to communicate so thoroughly that she can explain the same thing in various ways. If she fully understands an idea, a skill, or a problem, she will be able to communicate what she knows to the highly educated sophisticate as well as to the migrant worker with a language barrier.

The number and length of planned teaching sessions depend on the attention span of the patient. This ability will change as his health or medical condition changes. Long sessions with a toxic patient are futile, and do not contribute to the overall goal of nursing care. As the patient begins to recover, he begins to look outside of the restricted world where his major concern was his pain or disturbed health. He begins to notice his surroundings more, and becomes able to question and actually hear what is said.

In teaching, the nurse must know the *what* (content), the *how* (method), and in terms of the patient, she must know the *when*-ready (motivation). His readiness to learn is dependent on his physical and emotional ability to accept what the nurse teaches.

Emotions can enhance or hinder learning. The nurse will be more aware of the emotional overtones if she encourages responses or a continuing interchange during the teaching.

Social levels and ethnic origin can enhance or hinder learning. The beliefs of the patient must be understood by the nurse before she can expect to see success from her teaching. The patient's hearing may be good and his physical condition may show marked improvement, but he simply will not hear the directions for a procedure

TEACHING

or see its demonstration if he believes it is socially unacceptable. A case in point would be a urinary drainage bag for a permanent nephrostomy tube. There is a sex differential in the acceptance of the drainage bag—men seem to adjust more easily than do women, perhaps because a bag strapped to the leg of a man is more easily hidden than a bag fitted near the hip of a woman. As fashion changes, so may patient acceptance. Tight trousers could cause male patients difficulty, and fuller skirts could make the drainage bag more acceptable to women. The nurse must be aware of the impact of the outside world on the patient and help him make the adaptations necessary for his return to it.

The teaching process is applicable to the nursing care of all patients. Teaching is done in the hospital, home, clinic, school, and in industry. Though some content is vital to all patients, there is content that is especially important to the long-term patient, that concerns him more than other patients. This specific content includes: knowledge of the policies and rules of the hospital; the expected course of the disease process; reasons for procedures and activities; knowledge of community resources; and general health measures.

The long-term patient must be helped to know and understand what the policies and rules of the hospital or health agency are. The hospital becomes a home to him for a month or longer. Ease of adjustment is possible only if the expectations of the staff are made explicit to him. Any apparent confusion, or seeming lack of agreement among the staff add to the patient's stress and delay his recovery. He needs answers to such questions as: What are the usual routines? When are visitors permitted? When are meals served? Can I keep my own robe? Where are the bathrooms? When can I use the phone? What time must I go to bed? What time will the lights be put out? When should I expect my medicine?

The role the patient has in the hospital is a specific one, but no one bothers to tell him what it is. Too frequently the patient learns of the existence of a rule only after he has broken it. Such unplanned learning must be avoided. It is vital to the general well-being and eventual recovery of the patient that he be introduced early to the hospital setting, the staff, and to other patients.

If the patient is to be an intelligent reporter of his symptoms, he must know what to expect from the disease process. Instructions help the patient understand the disease, its course and limitations. The family should also be included, as they can be of assistance to the patient in learning ways and means of individual self-help.[8] The learning then becomes a family process.

There are patients who are unable to accept any information regarding their diagnosis or treatment. The nurse must be sensitive enough to learn this in her contacts with such patients. She must respect the wishes of the physician, the patient, and his family in regard to the disease specifics that she may discuss. However, as regards the patient who is approachable, the more he knows about his disease, the more he can see the importance of procedures and treatments he is expected to continue at home.

When the nurse demonstrates the procedures or treatments, she must explain their purpose to the patient. For example: Why are the irrigations important? Will they decrease symptoms? Will they stop pain? Will they keep a patient out of the hospital? A patient may ask: What is the use of that terrible-tasting medicine I have to take four times a day? Why do I have to learn to give myself shots; can't I take pills instead? Answering such questions by giving reasons based on knowledge is considerably more satisfying

TEACHING

to the patient than to be told to take a medicine because the doctor ordered it.

Patients need to learn to recognize signs of recovery and danger signals. Some patients will want to know the classification of the disease—where they stand in relation to others with the same disease. It may be useful in preventing further attacks for the patient to know how the disease started, its etiology.

Information about the specifics of a disease, its etiology, classification, epidemiology, and process, is widely available in medical texts, and a selection of these is accessible to any nurse. The patient needs the information, and the nurse is the one to bring it to him. The information must be accurate and up to date. Remember, the nurse is trying to overcome misconceptions; she must not compound them as happened in the case of the diabetic patient who was taught to boil his syringe and did so—but *after* the injection!—whereupon the syringe was stored in a cardboard box for the next use.[9] This could have been prevented if the nurse had carefully questioned the patient and listened.

In the medical sciences, facts become dated quickly. What is a marvel of a cure one year becomes a dangerous toxic agent the next. Thus, continued reading and checking of the newer drugs and treatments is basic to patient teaching.

Adequate follow-up and a knowledge of the vital part community resources play in providing for continuity of care are matters to be taught. As the patient knows more about his disease and the importance of continued health supervision, more responsibility must be assumed by the nurse in the hospital setting to make continuity of care a reality. A valuable adjunct to the nurse's ability to make adequate referrals is a knowledge of the local Directory of Social Agencies. This is most easily obtained through a public health nursing sequence in the nurse's educational preparation or experience. The Directory lists all of the social and health agencies in the community, giving location, intake policies, fees, hours, and extent of services. Looking over the directory of social agencies is an excellent way to begin an orientation to a new community. Many hospitals have an Inter-Agency Referral Form. If one does not, a phone call to the agency involved will clarify what type of information is vital to providing continuity of care. The content of the referral should be discussed with the patient. We often underestimate the benefit of joint planning and referral.

General health measures are the most difficult to teach. This is a broader and less specific area than procedures, treatments, disease patterns, and policies. For the long-term patient, general health measures become, in a sense, part of the treatment pattern. Information on bathing, cleanliness, and general diet can be shared easily during daily contacts. Often established health habits can be questioned, and with supportive teaching, a behavior change can occur.

Teaching becomes difficult when there are health habits the patient must change in order to survive. It is not so much teaching facts that is needed as assisting the patient to put health measures he already knows into practice—a most difficult task, as has already been mentioned. A common example of the need for change in behavior can be seen in the diabetic. The normal person can deviate widely from the principles of nutrition and not suffer immediate consequences. The cause-effect for the normal person is spread out in time. The diabetic does not have time as a buffer. This is why it is often easier to teach for survival rather than to teach for general improvement of health.

REFERENCES

1. Moore, Mary Lou, Staff Nursing Is Teaching Too. *American Journal of Nursing. 66:* 10, Oct. 1966. p. 2244.
2. Storlie, Frances J., This I Believe . . . About Who Shall Teach. *Nursing Outlook. 15:* 1, Jan. 1967. p. 53.
3. Pohl, Margaret L., *The Teaching Function of the Nursing Practitioner.* Dubuque, Iowa: Wm. C. Brown. 1968. 121 pp.
4. Vavaro, Filomena Fanelli, Teaching the Patient about Open Heart Surgery. *American Journal of Nursing. 65:* 10, Oct. 1965. p. 115.
5. Peplau, Hildegard, E., *Interpersonal Relations in Nursing.* New York: G.P. Putnam's Sons. 1952. 330 pp.
6. Rogers, Carl Ransom, *Client-Centered Therapy.* Boston: Houghton Mifflin. 1951. 572 pp.
7. Reik, Theodor, *Listening with the Third Ear.* New York: Farrar, Straus. 1949. 528 pp.
8. MacGinniss, Oscia, Rheumatoid Arthritis—My Tutor. *American Journal of Nursing. 68:* 8, Aug. 1968. pp. 1699-1701.
9. Watkins, Julia D., and Fay T. Moss,Confusion in the Managment of Diabetes *American Journal of Nursing. 69:* 3, March 1969. pp. 521-524.

7 COUNSELING

The long-term patient lives in a complex of interpersonal relationships. During the course of his life he has related to many people: his parents, spouse, children, friends, and work associates. Now that he is a patient, he has relationships with additional people: other patients, doctors, nurses, and other professional and nonprofessional workers. All will affect him—some positively, some negatively, and some neutrally. Engaging the active participation and cooperation of these people in the patient's therapeutic regime and coordinating his nursing care with other professional services comprise the counseling component of care.

The patient's need for counseling varies. The nurse must be aware of this and must have a sense of timing. Counseling should begin when the patient first comes into contact with the nurse. Most commonly this occurs in the doctor's office. The initial stages of a long-term illness, or the time during which it is being detected, are difficult for the patient and greatly influence future stages of his progress. Providing emotional support to the patient's spouse and/or family, at the time diagnostic tests are done, may make it possible for the spouse or family to return that support to the patient. Even if the family relationships are stable, the stress of a long-term illness will adversely affect the family members. If the family relationships are initially weak, the additional stress may precipitate total disintegration of the family unit.[1,2] If an acute exacerbation of an illness requires hospitalization, the patient and the family have many major problems. The adjustment to hospitalization is as great for the family as for the patient. A certain adaptability on the part of the hospital (such as allowing a husband to visit his wife outside of visiting hours because he works during those hours) will help in the adjustment. Also, preparations for any adjustment in home living patterns should begin during this first hospitalization, e.g., a change in family meal planning for a father hospitalized with cardiovascular renal disease. When the patient moves from the hospital back into his home, major nursing problems may continue or new ones may develop. Since very few patients have a nurse in their home 24 hours a day, active participation in nursing care and a good understanding of it is required of a family member. The patient who has moved from home to hospital and back to home has completed the typical cycle of nurse-patient contact; he is now again in contact with the office nurse or clinic nurse. At each point of the cycle, the nurse must be alert to the counseling needs of the patient, and be prepared and willing to fulfill them.

Counseling is the only component of care in which the focus of the nurse is shifted from the patient to other people in the patient's life, or from the one-to-one nurse-patient relationship to relationships which the nurse has with other people who are affecting the nursing care of the patient. This extension of relationships can be of two types. One engages others to participate actively in specific aspects of the nursing care of the patient. The second type coordinates nursing care with other professional services in order to create a total therapeutic atmosphere for the patient. The nurse may be engaged in both types of counseling simultaneously for the same patient, or for different patients. In either case the nurse is involved with others for the benefit of the patient.

Delegation of specific nursing responsibilities

In the nursing care of the long-term patient there are many instances when the nurse, personally, cannot meet each specific nursing need of the patient. The following situations illustrate the necessity of engaging someone else to participate in specific activities within each of the components of patient care.

Observations. Mr. Brown has just been diagnosed a diabetic and put on a diabetic regime. Though he is a vigorous man, he is in his seventies and shows some of the signs of senility, including forgetfulness. His housekeeper is the only person who can assume the hour-by-hour responsibility of observing for shock or coma. This specific nursing function can be taught to the housekkeeper either in the doctor's office, the patient's home, or during hospitalization.

Teaching. Mary Smith is a tuberculous teen-ager who has been intermittently hospitalized for treatment since the age of eight years. She lives with her divorced mother and two younger brothers. Mary knows well the course of her illness, its onset, its etiology, its communicability, but this is not enough; Mary's mother must be included in the teaching-learning process if any progress is to be expected. Keeping regular follow-up clinic appointments, guiding Mary's activities and diet, protecting the younger children from the disease, preventing future exacerbations and yet being prepared for them, are a few of the things Mrs. Smith must know how to do if Mary's nursing care plan is to be realized. The teaching can take place in the hospital, the clinic, or the home.

Emotional care. Mr. Moore is dying in a ward of elderly patients. He says he has lived his life and is ready to die, but he wants to discuss his impending death with someone. Since the one registered nurse on the floor is taking care of a new post-operative patient, the non-professional workers are the only ones who are available to fill Mr. Moore's emotional needs. If they have had guidance from the registered nurse in listening to a patient discuss death, Mr. Moore's emotional needs will probably be well met.

Physical care. Mr. Jones is home after having been hospitalized for a cardiovascular renal disease. He is bedridden 24 hours a day and has a visiting nurse who comes into the home once a week to bathe him and to give the meralluride injection. Between the visiting nurse's visits, Mrs. Jones takes care of her husband. The prevention of foot drop can be accomplished only if Mrs. Jones knows how to keep the foot board properly positioned and the top sheet and blanket pleated.

Treatment. Miss Meyer, a multiple sclerosis patient, lives at home with her mother. She and her family were once wealthy but they spent most of their money seeking a "cure." She refuses "charity" (i.e., county financed) hospitalization, although this will eventually be the only answer to her problem. Meanwhile, Miss Meyer has no bladder control and needs an indwelling catheter. A public health nurse comes into the home once a week to assist in Miss Meyer's physical care and to do a bladder irrigation and instillation. Because of the potential urinary complications and the daily needs for attention required by anyone having an indwelling catheter, Miss Meyer's mother must assume, under the guidance and supervision of the nurse, the responsibility for the care of the catheter between the nurse's visits.

Economics. Mrs. Robinson, 62 years of age, had lived with the condition of congestive heart failure and has had to maintain a restricted diet for many years. Her disease progressed to the point where her husband had to take over the shopping, cooking, and general housework. While the disease progressed, the Robinsons' fixed income decreased in purchasing power. The Robinsons needed help not only in over-all budgeting but also in the planning, purchasing, and preparing of foods. The most important nursing activity needed, according to the Robinsons, was assistance in "making the money stretch."

Correlated complexities. Mrs. Long, age 56, was in the hospital for amputation of the left leg due to gangrene resulting from a basic diabetic condition. When the family came to visit Mrs. Long, the nurse recalled that, though the cause of diabetes is unknown, a familial relationship exists in the incidence of the disease. Questioning Mrs. Long's daughter, a mother of three children, she found that the daughter was married to a man whose father had had diabetes. The nursing responsibilities here extended to case-finding. The nurse's advice that the daughter have her children periodically checked for diabetes resulted from a good understanding of the complexities of certain long-term illnesses.

These cases illustrate that no nurse can give all of the specific nursing care by herself in all situations. How often the nurse says, "But I did everything *I* could!" Yet the patient may need nursing care when the nurse herself is unavailable. At such times the delegation of specific responsibilities to others will help the patient receive the maximum benefit from the total nursing plan of care.

Working with the health team

Promotion of a therapeutic atmosphere by coordinating nursing care with other professional services is the other type of counseling. This is commonly known as working with the health team.

The health team has been defined in many different ways by many different authorities.[3] For the purposes of this book, it can be described as two or more people who are working together with the patient for his benefit. It can be an extensive team including patient, doctor, nurse, social worker, pharmacist, dietitian, occupational therapist, clergy, and ancillary personnel. The make-up of the team depends on the specific needs of the patient and the unique contribution each member of the team can make to his total care. The health team can be subdivided into smaller teams such as the nursing team and the medical team. The former includes professional nurses, practical nurses, nurses' aides—those directly responsible for the nursing care of the patient. The medical team includes only medical personnel. Ideally, the team consists of those persons who can help the patient achieve his maximum capacity for life with as much independence, comfort, dignity, and freedom from anxiety and pain as possible.

The purpose of the team is to provide, and to blend harmoniously, the various services which the patient needs. The initial team members have the responsibility for assessing the needs of the patient, for sharing their independent observations, appraisals, and judgments, and for establishing an overall plan of care. The need for ongoing, preplanned, and scheduled team conferences cannot be overemphasized. After the original planning session, team conferences can serve a number of functions: to keep each worker aware of his own contributions and responsibilities, to provide a direct method of communication among the team members, to evaluate the patient's progress toward the overall goal, to alter the original goal as circumstances may indicate, and to engage the services of other professional workers when the need arises. The nature of long-term illness implies that continuous, periodic re-evaluation and assessment are essential in the total care of the patient. For example, a 54-year-old man who is a devout Catholic is diagnosed initially as having cancer of the rectum. After hospitalization, he is re-diagnosed as having a terminal metastatic cancer. At this point, the health team needs to reformulate the patient's plan of care, decide when and who will tell the patient and his family of his impending death and how best to prepare the family for the patient's progressive deterioration and the care that will be required. They may make a decision about involving the parish priest if he has not been actively included before.

The three major factors that influence the functioning of any health team are: the personal needs of team members, time, and previous experience of the members with the team approach.

The focus of the health team is often clouded because the members use the team to perpetuate their own image or to meet their own personal needs. This can delay or block completely the realization of the goals of the patient's overall plan of care. Only when the focus of each team member is upon the patient and his family can the team approach be therapeutically successful.

"It takes time!" "Just a bit more time and everything will work out!" How often are such remarks excuses for personal inadequacies. On the other hand, how rarely is time given its proper importance in interpersonal relationships. The time necessary for the development of working relationships among members of the team may not only be overlooked but may even be considered nonessential. Yet any two people coming into contact with each other require *some* time for the development of a working relationship. The time can be shortened by self-understanding and a working knowledge of group processes.

Previous experience that team members may have had with the team approach can contribute much to their effectiveness. A successful experience reinforces the ability to engage in a similar experience. But how many successful health teams are functioning in the country today? And how accessible are the well-functioning teams to those seeking team experience? There are very few such teams and very few opportunities. At this point in history nurses have three alternatives: 1) to seek experience in recognized programs which include good team functioning, 2) to become familiar with descriptions in the literature of the team approach where it is working well, and 3) to engage in self-education through trial-and-error in developing successful health team experiences.

The team approach to patient care has evolved because the multiplicity of patient needs has resulted in a multiplicity of services. Each service is a professional entity, requiring knowledge, skills, and techniques of its members. No one service can solve all of the patient's problems. No one service can function independently in giving even minimal care to the patient.

The nurse needs broad knowledge and many skills in order to counsel and work well with others. She needs a sound understanding of the components of care to be able to adapt that care to the needs of a specific patient. She must develop the ability to realistically assess the capabilities of others whom she engages in specific nursing activities for the patient. When working with a family unit or a team, she must know about groups, their functioning and processes, and develop the ability to put this knowledge into practice. She needs a clear understanding of her role as a nurse, her professional responsibilities and limitations. She must be able to communicate to others what her role is and to fulfill it.

REFERENCES

1. Parsons, Talcott, and Renee C. Fox, Illness, Therapy and the Modern Urban American Family, in *A Modern Introduction to The Family*. Norman W. Bell and Ezra F. Vogel, Eds. New York: The Free Press. 1966. pp. 346-360.
2. Levy, Marion J. Jr., Aspects of the Analysis of Family Structure, in *Aspects of the Analysis of Family Structure*. Ansley J. Coale, Lloyd A. Fallers, Marion J. Levy, Jr., David M. Schneider, and Silvan S. Tomkins. Princeton, New Jersey: Princeton University Press. 1965. p. 59.
3. Coulter, Pearl Parvin, *The Nurse in the Public Health Program*. New York: G. P. Putnam's Sons. 1954. pp. 3-31.

8 ECONOMICS

Poverty and long-term illness go hand in hand in American society. The onset and progression of a long-term illness are accompanied by an increase in expenditures and a decrease in earning power. The nurse who has not personally experienced the costs of a long-term illness may find the economics of disability difficult to comprehend. The following example shows the economic effect of a long-term illness upon an ordinary middle-income family.

Mr. Marr was a successful automobile salesman. He lived in a three-bedroom house in the suburbs with his wife and two children. With $500 saved for emergencies and with hospital expense protection and adequate life insurance policies, they felt quite secure. The payments on their house and car were within their budget.

At the age of 43, Mr. Marr suffered a serious head injury in a car accident and had to undergo neurosurgery. The medical expenses very quickly used up the Marrs' financial resources. Their immediate expenses included ambulance cost, hospital bill, physician's fee, neurosurgeon's fee, special duty nurse's fee, and other costly items. The health insurance that they carried was limited and insufficient.

Mrs. Marr went to work and assumed the role of the family breadwinner. As a woman and an unskilled laborer, her earnings were less than Mr. Marr's had been. While the family income decreased, living expenses increased. With the mother of the family working away from home, the cost of a baby sitter had to be added to the budget. Since Mrs. Marr had less time for cooking, the food bill went up. Transportation expenses increased because Mrs. Marr had to use the family car to go both to work and to the hospital to see her husband. The family sold their house and moved to a cheaper place, spending what the sale brought them on the mounting medical costs.

Mr. Marr recovered with a partial paralysis. He came home from the hospital, but the expense of a long-term illness continued. Mr. Marr needed weekly physical therapy for two years. He required close, continual medical supervision. His nutritional needs were more expensive after the accident than before. He needed the part-time services of a visiting nurse at home. His partial paralysis and impaired speech prevented him from returning to his job. The office of vocational rehabilitation in his state declared him "totally disabled." The lower standard of living continued for the family.

Yet in the national picture of long-term illness the Marr family was lucky. Though their total pattern of living was changed, Mrs. Marr was able to assume the financial responsibilities and the role of head of the family. The average American family cannot possibly afford a long-term illness. For most, it is hard enough to pay for the acute illnesses which occur.

The economic hardships and difficulties of meeting the costs of a long-term illness have led to the development of sources that can help defray the medical costs. These include: voluntary health insurance; workmen's compensation; industrial and union medical care programs; non-occupation disability insurance; old-age and survivors' insurance; public assistance programs; philanthropic agencies; and payments by life insurance, group accidental death and dismemberment insurance, personal accident insurance, and liability insurance.

Each of these have been identified and defined by the Commission on Chronic Illness.[1] None is designed specifically to assist the long-term patient. Though all pay for some medical costs, none are adequate to meet all the costs of a long-term illness. The major limitations relate to eligibility for assistance, types and amounts of benefits available, and the coordination of local, regional, and national services.

The advent of national legislation, in the form of Public Law 89-97 (1965), has changed the economic effects of a long-term illness for one segment of the population, namely, those citizens over 65 years of age.[2] As Robert Ball has written, ". . . because of Medicare, many more elderly Americans have been able to get hospital care with the dignity that goes with the ability to pay . . ."[3] (The effect of Medicare upon nursing services can be found in References 4, 5, 6, 7, and 8.)

The distressing fact is that the age group of 20 to 65, which is the backbone of American society, has not only the highest incidence of long-term illness, but the least financial resources for meeting it. The increase in medical care costs in the last few years, according to the Department of Health, Education and Welfare, has been due to population increase, inflationary pressures in the economy, wider insurance coverage, and the conviction that every American should have access to quality medical care.

Whatever the national scene is, the nurse has certain responsibilities in the sphere of economics when caring for the long-term patient. Her awareness of the problem and its effect upon the patient's condition, his family, and the well-being of all, is first and foremost. In our culture a person will readily discuss the price of his car, his annual income, or the costs of education. He is reticent, however, about discussing his financial problems. Admitting that one lacks money would seem to be equivalent to admitting that one is inadequate. The long-term patient is by definition in a dependent position—one who is unable to care for his daily needs. The mere presence of a nurse is an admission of inadequacy in one sphere of life, namely health. Therefore, it is difficult for a patient to discuss financial worries, thus admitting inadequacy in another sphere of life, economics. The sensitive nurse weighs her knowledge of the patient, assesses the reality of his financial worries, and then discusses the situation with the patient. The nurse's attitude must be non-judgmental (the attitude discussed in the chapter on Emotional Support). Because of the closeness which is inherent in the nurse-patient relationship, the nurse is in an optimal position to pick up clues regarding present and potential financial problems. It is her duty to elicit information from the patient, and to do it tactfully. The action to be taken upon gaining the information may be a referral to a social worker, an insurance adjuster, or a doctor; or it may consist merely in the nurse remaining a sympathetic listener.

The activity of referral, the liaison function between the patient and other persons, is common practice in nursing. (A good guide to referral systems, the process, the philosophy, and some suggested forms, is found elsewhere.[9]) The importance of a timely referral in caring for a long-term patient is incalculable. A referral to a social worker about the patient's financial problems may simplify and hasten the treatment of his medical condition. A referral, made jointly with the physician, to a local Heart Association for an evaluation of the patient's work capacity may assist him to maintain his independence and his capacity as an economically productive member of the community.

The activity of referral is based upon a knowledge of available sources of financial assistance and vocational rehabilitation. This knowledge begins with the fact that sources of assistance vary from community to community, from state to state, and from region to region. The only constant financial source is national aid, such as Old-Age and Survivors' Insurance. It is the individual nurse's responsibility to be aware of the existing resources; she may do this through in-service education, or through professional associations and activities.

The socio-economic problems of long-term illness cannot be solved in the nurse-patient relationship. However, the nurse does contribute to the solution of the problems as a member of the nursing profession and as a citizen who has voting rights and responsibilities. In the nurse-patient relationship the nurse must assume some responsibilities for the economic problems revolving around the patient's physical problems, but direct financial aid to the patient or the family is not among those responsibilities.

Direct aid is the function of other health-workers, both in voluntary organizations like the American Cancer Society, and in public agencies like the Bureau of Public Assistance. The responsibilities of the nurse include an awareness and understanding of the patient's financial problems, the activity of referral, the knowledge of sources of assistance, and the teaching of basic budget planning and of savings possible through conservation of materials.

In the crises of a long-term illness, when expenditures mount so rapidly, the ability to cut costs safely is invaluable to a family. The nurse can teach basic budgeting to the family, particularly in the patient's home, and help the family cut their living expenses. To give just one example of saving safely: the cost of powdered milk is approximately one-fourth the cost of fresh milk. Powdered milk can be palatable if mixed with a rotary beater and chilled overnight. The nutritional values of powdered milk and fresh milk are the same, except for the fat content. In a family with children who need large quantities of milk, the use of powdered milk is nutritionally sound and relatively inexpensive.

The principles of teaching budgeting are the same as those discussed in the chapter on teaching. The knowledge required is that of current market costs and the needs of the patient. An elderly patient with anemia, no teeth, and living on Social Security cannot afford to buy canned baby foods, nor can he be expected to relish their taste.

Equipment, drugs, and dressings are costly. The nurse in any setting is the prime user and dispenser of these items. Their cost is obscured to the hospital nurse who is not responsible for billing, fees, and the hospital budget. Ordering supplies from central supply may be a clerical task to the nurse, but she must be careful in doing so; each item used is one more hospital expense to the patient. Well-organized and supervised care in the preparation for and management of costly laboratory tests which the patient may need will expedite their conclusion without the expensive necessity of having to repeat them. Securing and caring for equipment in a patient's home is another matter. Many times the nurse not only uses the equipment but is also responsible for advising the patient to purchase it and for supervising its care and maintenance. Most public health nurses are alert to the costs of equipment and are accustomed to helping patients improvise equipment. The field of improvisation of equipment for home care is amply covered in the literature.[10]

The cost of drugs is becoming an increasingly controversial subject. The difference in cost between ordering drugs by brand name or by generic name has been the topic of many journal articles. The nurse, if aware of the problem, can be a factor in reducing unnecessary drug costs to the patient through good professional working relationships with pharmacists and doctors.

Special equipment in patient care is one thing; personal and household equipment is another. Does the patient at home really need clean sheets each day? Can the elderly patient who has no washing machine afford to send his sheets to a laundry? (The nurse should make an actual check of local prices.) How thoughtless is the nurse and how expensive her service if she drops a staining medication on a patient's nylon nightgown! The nurse strengthens the relationship with the long-term patient by demonstrating a concern for the costs of equipment, drugs, and dressings.

In the total picture of the economics of long-term illness, the extent of the nurse's activities and responsibilities is limited. They are, nevertheless, important in the care of the patient. The patient's financial worries can so adversely affect his therapeutic regime as to negate it entirely. Recognizing and attempting to help to treat the patient's financial ills are as important as treating his physical, emotional, or social ills.

REFERENCES

1. Commission of Chronic Illness, *Chronic Illness in the United States.* Vol. II, *Care of the Long-Term Patient.* Cambridge, Mass.: Harvard University Press. 1957. pp. 370-413.
2. United States Congress, *Public Law 89-97.* (89th Congress, H. R. 6675) 1965. 138 pp.

3. Ball, Robert M., After One Year, Medicare Accomplishments. *Nursing Outlook. 15:* 8, Aug. 1967. p. 47.
4. *Changes in Nursing Visit Load of Public Health Nursing Agencies, 1965-1967.* New York: National League for Nursing. 1969. 5 pp.
5. Candland, Louise, The Home Care Administrator. *Nursing Outlook. 16:* 1, Jan. 1968. pp. 30-33.
6. Tierney, Thomas M., The Continuing Partnership. *Nursing Outlook. 16:* 1, Jan. 1968. pp. 22-24.
7. Griffith, Elsie I., Where Do V.N.A.'s Go from Here? *Nursing Outlook. 16:* 3, March 1968. pp. 29-31.
8. Pope, Irene, Medicare—Impetus for Change. *Nursing Outlook. 16:* 1, Jan. 1968. pp. 34-35.
9. Joint Committee of Integration of Social and Health Aspects of Nursing in the Basic Curriculum, Referral of Patients for Continuity of Care. *Public Health Nursing. 39,* 1947. pp. 568-573.
10. American Red Cross, *Home Nursing Textbook.* New York: Doubleday. 1951. pp. 135-217.

9 COMPLEX CORRELATIONS

The nurse needs considerable knowledge to care for the long-term patient. She draws her knowledge from the sciences and from her experience. Further knowledge derives from the intertwining of two or more groups of knowledge. Knowledge of such correlations is a component of nursing which can improve its practice and thereby aid the patient in his recovery.* Correlations have been observed in practice, and they are reported in increasing numbers in the literature. The examples cited here should not be viewed as independently valuable—they are cited to demonstrate patterns or, as we call them, complex correlations. Such correlations will emerge with any large sampling of the literature or organization of one's varied experience. The correlations may occasionally be stated explicitly by a particular study, or a group of studies may suggest that a non-specified factor may be operative in each of these several studies. Reading, observing, and thinking help the nurse discover patterns or correlations.

---

* The term correlation is used here as in statistics, though no correlation coefficients are reported. Correlation between two or more factors means that they occur together—when one factor is present the other factor is also present. No cause-effect relationship is established. The causative agent may be quite distinct and separate from the two or more factors which are correlated.

How valid and scientific are these correlations? The nurse must be able to answer this question in order to prevent misapplication or inaccurate thinking. Observed correlations are partially dependent on the quality of the observation. However, even when given a high quality of observation, there is a marked difference between the knowledge based on a statistical significance of factors and a cause-effect relationship which can be repeatedly shown. Proof is absent in the bulk of medical writing today. An historical example of the systematic building up of evidence that leads to an inescapable conclusion (or-proof) is the work of Robert Koch on the tubercle bacillus.[1] There is, however, a certain utility in careful studies even though the element of proof is lacking. Nurses must learn to see how the quality of studies varies and must learn to judge the appropriateness of methods used in the investigation of certain types of problems. To become intelligent consumers of research, nurses should seek this necessary preparation in universities and colleges.

Much has been written on psychosomatic diseases. There does seem to be a correlation between the patient's personality, the defense mechanisms he uses, and the presence of certain diseases. Unfortunately, the emphasis on the role that emotions play in illness often leads the nurse to discount the importance of a psychosomatic disease. It must be remembered that *every* patient, no matter what the origins of his disease are, needs care, relief from pain, and sensitive concern from a knowledgeable nurse.

There are multiple factors that are related to the presence of disease. In addition to the contribution of the individual's personality, there are external factors in the patient's life pattern, familial factors and socio-economic and ethnic factors. The following examples illustrate these multiple factors.

The severity of rheumatoid arthritis seems to be proportionate to the severity of the impairment in the capacity to express aggression.

The illness of patients with tuberculosis has been observed to occur during states of exhaustion that followed failure of defensive mechanisms.

Many chronic disease patients report a feeling of helplessness and hopelessness immediately preceding the onset of the symptoms of the illness which led to hospitalization. Either a real or threatened loss of a love object has been implicated in the precipitation of cancer, tuberculosis, rheumatoid arthritis, congestive heart failure, and other conditions.

Patients hospitalized for treatment of tuberculosis who left the hospital before completing their treatment have more problems in relation to loneliness and feelings of isolation than do patients who remain in the hospital for total treatment. It has been observed that stress, such as accompanies the first few weeks of attending medical school or important final examinations, is accompanied by a significant rise in cholesterol level. Stress, particularly in relation to occupation, has frequently been implicated in tuberculous male patients leaving the hospital before their disease has been adequately treated.

Lack of affection and attention from the mother is reported to explain difficulties in sexual identification and adjustment of women with rheumatoid arthritis.

Medical students with hypertensive parents have been shown to be more reactive to cigarette smoking than students with normal parents. Circulatory response to smoking in the healthy young adult strongly suggests that it depends in part upon the physiological heritage of the individual. There is a greater incidence of rheumatoid arthritis in relatives of rheumatoid individuals than in the general population.

There is a positive relationship between the mortality from arteriosclerotic heart disease and population density. Possibly the difference in living rather than in diet is the etiological factor of arteriosclerotic heart disease. Stated another way, the higher the income the less likely a death, the lower the income the more likely a death from coronary disease.

The economic level of an area or nation may have an influence on the possibility of decreasing or eradicating tuberculosis. Both positive and negative influences of economics toward the control of tuberculosis have been reported from widely scattered areas such as the Bahamas, Brazil, India, and Tanganyika.

There are ethnic influences. For example, in New York, cervical cancer is lowest in Jewish women, higher in non-Jewish whites, higher in Negro women, and highest in Puerto Rican women.

Other countries report similar influences of race. An ethnic difference was noted in a tuberculin survey of children in Kuwait. The Kuwaiti children showed the lowest incidence of positive reactions to the tuberculin compared with the Lebanese and other non-Kuwaiti. However, the Kuwaiti children showed the highest incidence of active pulmonary tuberculosis, suggesting that they are less resistant to the disease than the non-Kuwaitis.

The factors just noted direct the nurse's awareness to the fact that the development of illness is indeed due to more than a single organism or to a "negative personality." It is also important to recognize that the reverse of the psychosomatic disease is true. The body influences the mind and the mind influences the health of the body. Because it is quite difficult to be sure when disease is implicated in personality changes, the confused patient should not be immediately labeled as "senile" or "disoriented." Rather, the nurse should consider that his confusion may be due to any number of factors. Impairment in the circulation of the brain, for instance, rapidly results in confusion and behavior change. Change in cerebral circulation may be due to a variety of factors, such as disturbance of fluid and electrolyte balance, nutritional deprivation, anoxia, or hypoxia. The fluid and electrolyte balance at times may be resolved with a careful watching of the intake and output of fluids. The anoxia may be resolved by an adjustment in the respirator.

Part of the difficulty the nurse experiences in relating the complex correlations is due to the commonly held theory of dichotomy of body and mind, the psyche and the soma. But the individual is a totality, and although we need to separate the systems for the purposes of learning structure and function, we must recognize the interdependence of the systems of body and mind.

Even when internal or external factors and disease are separated, one can note that patterns occur in diseases that affect the long-term patient. Some diseases occur together more frequently than do others. It is rare to see a patient with both rheumatoid arthritis and asthma, but common to see a patient with a peptic ulcer and rheumatoid arthritis. The peptic ulcer may have existed prior to any treatment for the arthritis, though it has been shown that peptic ulcers frequently result from cortisone treatment of arthritis.

The chart on page 100 is a summary of conditions that occur together. The chart is limited to the major chronic illnesses, e.g., arthritis, tuberculosis, cancer, and cardiovascular disease.

Correlations Between Diseases, Conditions, or Therapy

Arthritis	Cancer	Heart and Vascular	Tuberculosis	
+	+	+	+	cardiovascular disease
+	+	+	+	renal disease
+	+	+	+	neoplasms
+	+	+	+	pulmonary changes
+	+	0	0	untoward effects of radiation therapy
+	+	0	+	duodenal ulcers and/or chronic gastritis
+	+	+	+	nutritional deficiency
+	+	+	0	endocrine disturbance
+	0	+	0	obesity
+	0	+	0	rheumatoid, collagen disease
0	+	+	+	anemia
0	0	+	+	diabetes
0	+	+	0	hypertension
0	+	0	0	cirrhosis
0	+	0	+	silicosis

\+ = known to exist together frequently
0 = no reported frequent relationship

In addition to the pattern in the chart, there are other diseases or conditions that occur together with only one of the above listed diseases as, for example, chronic irritation and poor hygiene with penile cancer. Alcoholism, recently classified and treated as a disease, is frequently associated with tuberculosis.

Problems multiply for the patient who has more than one disease. Nursing care is complicated and both diagnosis and treatment become difficult. Some of the adverse interactions between drugs have been noted in the chapter on treatment. Certain drugs are metabolized by enzyme action and the by-products may be toxic. Phenobarbital, for example, stimulates the enzyme that metabolizes dicoumarol. The sedation may be effective, but the anticoagulant effect is reduced. Biochemical toxicity may occur in the patient who is taking certain antidepressant drugs and who eats cheese at the same time.

The intertwining of diseases and conditions can lead to difficulty in treatment and management. The classical textbook picture of a disease becomes clouded, and the specified technique may be difficult to apply, when a patient has multiple problems. Awareness of such correlations will help the nurse in adapting techniques rather than continuing them without variation when the situation warrants a change.

Regrouping the complex correlations into two broad classifications for discussion may simplify the approach. Rather than looking at the patient's personality and his social and ethnic background separately, the following organization can be used:

1. *Factors associated with the precipitation or extension of the disease.*

2. *Factors that do not seem to contribute directly to the onset of the disease, but that are frequently associated with the disease.*

These factors will be discussed side by side.

Stress* is a precipitating factor for many chronic diseases. It is stress in the form of a real or threatened loss.

---

* The theory of stress proposed by Hans Selye[2,3] continues to be controversial but demands attention. Dr. Selye was able to demonstrate repeatable physiological response to stress. The three stages of the General Adaptation Syndrome (G.A.S.) or stress syndrome are: 1) alarm reaction, 2) stage of resistance, and 3) stage of exhaustion. The alarm reaction consists of adrenal enlargement, thymicolymphatic involution, and ulcers in the gastrointestinal tract. Loss of body weight may also occur. In the stage of resistance the manifestations are opposite to the alarm reaction. There is a rapid production of adrenocortical hormones, and the body tries to combat the factors causing stress. After prolonged exposure to stress, resistance falters, and exhaustion, the third stage of adaptation, begins. The symptoms are strikingly similar to those of the initial alarm reaction. The phenomenon is reversible, but if stress continues, death ensues.

Imperfections or imbalance of the G.A.S. are implicated in many of the chronic diseases for which no specific etiological agent is known.

Onset of symptoms occurs at the loss of a significant personal relationship. The stress is expressed in feelings of helplessness, hopelessness, and worthlessness together with anxiety and loss of self-esteem.

The stress factor may or may not be closely associated in time with the onset of symptoms. In some patients disease begins within a week after a severe personal loss. In others, separation or threat of separation occurs six months or more before the onset of the disease.

How the individual reacts to a specific stress depends on many factors. Sensitivity varies, but regardless of how adaptable an individual may be, it can be assumed that there are some forms of stress he can tolerate less than others. The determinants of susceptibility to illness are both genetic and environmental. The actual life situations encountered are less important than the way in which they are perceived. In some patients who have a particular disorder, stimulation of the sensory modality most closely related to that disorder arouses more emotional response than does stimulation of another modality. For example, the arthritic is more sensitive to muscle stimulation than the asthmatic, and the asthmatic is more sensitive to changes in olfactory stimulation than the arthritic.

Those with a *familial history* of a disease are more likely to get that disease. Higher, more labile blood pressure, faster heart-rate, and overweight, for instance, are more frequent among students whose parents had hypertension. There is definite evidence that primary hypertension occurs with greater frequency in some families than in others.

A new problem may be developing. Patients with congenital cardiac defects are now surviving and reproducing. There is evidence of second-generation congenital heart defects.

As already mentioned, one of the *socio-economic factors*

precipitating disease is the (relative) density of population. But cities are not necessarily the culprits. For example, contrary to what one would expect, the prevalance of rheumatic and congenital heart disease was found to be greater among rural than among urban dwellers in 41 counties in Colorado. The differences were best explained on the basis of environmental factors. It turned out there were more people per room in the rural areas than in the urban.

An ethnic factor, already mentioned, is the low rate of cervical cancer among Jewish women; this factor may be associated with circumcision. There is an even lower rate of cervical cancer among Jewish women who practice the Mosaic rule of abstinence from intercourse the week following their menses.

Socio-economic factors play a part in delaying the diagnosis of a condition. The specific factors are: social level, monetary consideration, anxiety over the possibility of a specific disease, personal negligence, negative attitudes toward medicine and hospitals, presence of defense mechanisms, superficiality of site of a disease, and lack of awareness of the seriousness of the implications of disease. Physicians who practice among the lower socio-economic groups, for example, tend to be more prompt in suspecting tuberculosis than physicians practicing among the upper socio-economic groups.

The unmarried, unskilled laborer has a higher incidence of disease than the married skilled laborer, and the impairments are more severe when present. Low income and low education are frequently associated with arthritis, cancer, tuberculosis, and heart disease. An interesting constellation of education and income is suggested by an extensive study of persons with rheumatoid arthritis. The incidence was higher where: 1) education was low and income high, and 2) education was high and income low. The discrepancy between education and income sets the stage for stress of many kinds, which in turn may precipitate the arthritis.

Indigency cannot be classified as precipitating disease as directly as stress, but disease definitely goes along with it. Multiple impairments are the rule rather than the exception for the indigent family. Most of the disabled persons from indigent families have been disabled for a long time, and in at least one-half of the cases the disability ranges from moderate to severe. Practically all have multiple chronic conditions, a high percentage of which are degenerative types of diseases and mental and emotional conditions.

Indigency tends to perpetuate itself even when patients are given the opportunity for vocational rehabilitation. One study showed that, following the inactivation of pulmonary tuberculosis, patients who were employed before hospitalization became employed in significantly higher numbers than patients who were on public assistance or pension before hospitalization.

There are some specific sociologic factors which have been associated with cardiovascular mortality rates in the last three decades. There is a difference in the rates for males and females. Urbanization, prosperity, and less activity have been more detrimental to men. The diet pattern of men has changed to more animal fats, while women have changed their dietary habits in order to retain a fashionably slim figure. Women have fewer children than formerly and can slow down at ages 40-60. Men have greater psychological stress in job situations, and the social structure has not encouraged them to slow down during the age range of 40 to 60.

There continues to be considerable controversy over high fat content in the diet as a factor associated with the presence of atherosclerosis and its complications. The relation has not definitely been established. It has been believed that the Orientals as a group were free from atherosclerosis because of their dietary habits. In an extensive study at thirteen university teaching hospitals in seven Oriental countries, the researchers found hypertension and atherosclerosis quite common, although varying in frequency and severity from place to place. Coronary and cerebral arterial disease was found everywhere. National habits regarding dietary fat cannot be considered as the sole or major etiological agent, for in some areas low intake of fat is associated with high incidence of disease. The presence of disease appears to be unrelated to the intake of salt or the influences of western civilization.

Another current controversy is the relation of air pollution to respiratory disease. Tobacco continues to be named as a potent pollutant of inspired air which contributes to respiratory disease.

Knowledge of specific facts is necessary for an understanding of a disease and the planning of nursing care. It is, however, unrealistic to consider a disease as being separate, well-defined, and existing alone. This outdated concept goes back to the germ theory, which, has been of great help to the health professions in the control of many diseases, but has also clouded the importance of other factors in the etiology and maintenance of disease. The inadequacy of the germ theory is particularly apparent in considering the major health problem in the United States today, that of chronic diseases, many of which have no known etiological agent.

REFERENCES

1. Koch, Robert, *The Aetiology of Tuberculosis.* Translated

by Dr. and Mrs. Max Pinner. New York: National Tuberculosis Assoc. 1932. 48 pp.
2. Selye, Hans, *The Physiology and Pathology of Exposure to Stress: a treatise based on the concepts of the general adaptation syndrome and the diseases of adaptation.* 1st edition. Montreal: Acta. 1950. 822 pp.
3. Selye, Hans, *The Stress of Life.* New York: McGraw-Hill. 1956. 324 pp.

10 DEATH, THE INEVITABLE: AN APPROACH

The nurse helps patients and their families meet many crises in life—birth, illness, disease, separation, loss, and death. Of these, the death of a patient is perhaps the most difficult event that the nurse and the family have to meet.

The nurse is a member of a profession that is a part of Western culture, a culture that regards death as a social taboo—as a life phenomenon that must be denied because it is unmeasurable by scientific parameters. Until 1968, when the American Nurses' Association Convention adopted the revised "Code for Nurses with Interpretive Statements," the nursing profession had reflected the Western traditions of denying and avoiding death. Part of the interpretation of the first statement of the Code reads*:

The nurse's respect for the worth and dignity of the individual human being extends throughout the entire life cycle, from birth to death, and is reflected in her care of the defective as well as the normal, the patient with a longterm in contrast to an acute illness, the young and the old, the recovering patient as well as the one who is terminally ill or dying. In the latter instance

* A deeper understanding of the nursing profession's stand on its responsibilities and obligations to the dying patient and to death can be obtained easily through a study of the evolution of the code of ethics. It begins with Isabel Hampton Robb's *Nursing Ethics* in 1909[1] and ends with the most recent "Code for Nurses with Interpretive Statements" in 1968.[2]

the nurse should use all the measures at her command to enable the patient to live out his days with as much comfort, dignity, and freedom from anxiety and pain as possible. His nursing care will determine, to a great degree, how he lives this final human experience and the peace and dignity with which he approaches death.[3]

It is commendable that the nursing profession has taken official steps to acknowledge the nurse's involvement with, and obligations to, patients and their families in the crises of death.

Any consideration of death must also deal with a new definition. When heart and other organ transplants became a part of surgical procedure, new professional problems appeared. It was to prevent the accusation of "body snatching" that the medical profession, in cooperation with other health professionals and with the clergy, discussed the issue and its ethical, moral, and legal implications. The definition of death as "irreversible brain death" has been discussed in the recent nursing literature.[4]

Death is a common occurrence in long-term illness nursing. Of the ten leading causes of death in 1967, seven were due to chronic conditions.*

Ten leading causes of death in USA in 1967[5]

Condition	Rate per 100,000 population
*Heart	364.5
*Malignant neoplasms	157.2
*Vascular lesions of CNS	102.2
Accidents	57.2
Diseases of infancy	24.4
Influenza, Pneumonia	28.8
*General arteriosclerosis	19.0
*Diabetes	17.7
*Other diseases of the circulatory system	15.1
*Other bronchopulmonic diseases	14.8

Five chronic conditions that contribute to the ten leading causes of death have increased in rate per 100,000 of the population since 1950.

Death rate of selected chronic conditions 1950, 1955, 1958, 1967[6]

Condition	Rate per 100,000 population			
	1950	1955	1958	1967
Heart	356.9	356.5	367.9	367.9
Malignant neoplasms	139.8	146.5	146.9	157.2
Vascular lesions of CNS	104.0	106.0	110.1	102.2
General arteriosclerosis	20.4	19.8	19.9	19.0
Diabetes	10.2	15.5	15.9	17.7

The preceding statistical tables indicate that the care of the dying patient commands considerable attention in the nursing care of the long-term patient. The quality of the care which a nurse can give is dependent upon the richness of her conceptualization. The components of care that are presented and developed in this book have application to every nursing situation, including that in which the nurse cares for the patient who is anticipating or meeting death. In order to illustrate this, incidents from the practice of individual nurses will be cited.[7] Regardless of the setting in which the following incidents occurred, the components of care in each are applicable in any setting.

The process of conceptualization

Death is difficult to face. I remember the first time I met it in nurses' training. Two of us were assigned to prepare the body of a patient who had died just before we came on duty. This happened on the men's medical ward of a county hospital where death was common and no one seemed to pay much attention to it. My classmate and I wrapped the body under the supervision of our nursing arts instructor who was extremely impersonal.

Obviously, we were expected to have no feelings—just follow explicitly the written 1-2-3-4 steps of the care-of-the-body-after-death procedure.

I knew better than to speak out, but my heart cried out. Doesn't this man have any family? Why did he have to die alone? Is he at peace now? Was he frightened? What kind of a man had he been? Had he lived a full life? His body was obviously old. Oh, why couldn't we talk about him and make all this less impersonal? I was upset—not at the death but at the way death was being handled. I pondered over death for a long time.

I met death often in those student days, but never satisfactorily. Regulations prohibited taking anyone's feelings into consideration. My heart ached for the families. They were allowed to be with the patient only ten minutes out of an hour if the doctors thought death was imminent. Or they were called at home, unprepared for the news, after the death, and allowed to view the body for a minute if they came to the hospital immediately. How little life seemed to matter, and how I inwardly rebelled against this.

I can look back now at this period and see it in the light of my later experiences and greater maturity. Even though I still feel the impersonal treatment of death was wrong, I can understand that reaction a little better. Death is a phenomenon that no one wants to face. By evading its personal effect and by treating it scientifically, one can attempt to keep one's emotional armor from being pierced. I am very glad, however, that my student days are over and that I can now react to nursing situations more as an individual and with my own feelings.

This nurse began by questioning the impersonality displayed by an instructor. The selection and organization of facts followed the questioning. Gradually she recognized a behavior change in herself. The process of conceptualization requires time and effort. It also requires a group of facts or content such as personal care, emotional care, and the other components of the care of the long-term patient.

The following sections are devoted to a presentation of content essential to giving excellent care to patients.

Observations

In observing the dying patient the most important sense is the sixth sense. A young nurse working the 3—11 shift on a surgical unit reported the following incident.

"I'm going to die. I want my wife." The man's skin was blanched, perspiration stood out on his forehead, and his pupils were large black dots.

"Are you having pain?" I asked.

"No, but I know this is it," he replied.

For a moment I was stunned. Die! But he isn't critical! I checked his vital signs immediately, and everything was within the normal range. The time was 7 p.m., and I remembered that at report in the afternoon the head nurse said he was three weeks postoperative and doing fine.

"Please," he pleaded, "I'm afraid. Don't leave me alone." The feeling of apprehension crept over me too.

In answer to his plea I said, "I won't leave you alone. I'm going to have the orderly stay with you while I call the doctor and your wife; and then I will come back."

After the orderly arrived I left the room with a feeling of confusion. All the physical signs did not point to death, yet he insisted he was dying.

The doctor was called and told of the patient's apprehension. The doctor gave permission to call the wife if the supervisor felt it was necessary. When the supervisor was asked, she came up to the patient's room. When she left the room a few minutes later, she brought out the orderly and said, "He will be fine now. I gave him a pep talk. There isn't any reason to call his wife. It's after visiting hours anyway."

Even though the supervisor seemed so sure, I couldn't dismiss my apprehension about the patient. Upon returning to the room I found him crying. "Why must I die alone? She won't call my wife. When my wife comes to get me, tell her that I love her very much and always will love her."

I immediately left the room and again called the supervisor, who finally consented to call the wife. I returned to the patient's room and told him that his wife had been called and that she would come soon.

The patient's wife arrived at 10 p.m. At midnight the patient died.

This example illustrates the importance of the sixth sense. Very little is known about a patient's awareness of impending death, but few people deny its existence. The nurse is crucial in detecting the patient's awareness and in acting appropriately upon her observation.

Physical care

The physical care of the dying patient requires of the nurse highly developed technical skills as well as ingenuity. How common is this report from one nurse to another:

> Mr. Jones, in Room 220, is in bad shape. The oxygen is going at 6 liters; Dr. Mann says keep it there. He fights the mask, so check the restraints to see that they are tight. He does a lot of muttering but don't let him get that mask off. The catheter is draining all right but his output is not too much. The second I.V. was started an hour ago because he hadn't been taking fluids. There's a third I.V. ordered. And don't let the needle get out of the vein whatever you do. There's another cath irrigation ordered for tonight. He has apparently got prostate trouble. The urine's cruddy. We pulled the covers tight to try to keep him quiet and warm. He's been tossing and turning all day.

is unwise to have pain medication on a prn pattern because this pattern places too much responsibility on the patient to ask for the medication. Rather, pain medication should be given regularly around the clock. In this manner, often smaller doses of the narcotic are needed.

A search for more pain-reducing medications needs to be made. The problem of depression resulting from the use of some pain-killing narcotics needs to be solved. An adaptation was made in England with the use of heroin.[12] This preparation, given under supervision, seems to cause less depression than do many other narcotics, and provides considerable relief from pain.

Teaching

A component of care can be minor in one nursing situation and paramount in another. In the care of the dying patient, teaching becomes a minor component. Even though a patient is semi-comatose, he often can hear and understand what is taking place within his room. The nurse should explain the "how" and "why" of any procedure. Such teaching does not lead to the end goal of behavior change; rather, it relates to and reinforces emotional support of the patient.

In the care of a patient whose condition is affected by the death of someone close to him, teaching the patient becomes a paramount component. For example, the mother of a child who dies at birth of multiple congenital anomalies should be told the truth about causes of congenital anomalies. Dispelling fears created by cultural patterns can readily contribute to the mother's recovery and future general health. Another example is the patient admitted with a diagnosis of tuberculosis who fears the disease because his father died of it. There are many instances in which the thought of death is a factor in a patient's situation, and in which his progress is dependent upon the teaching skills of the nurse.

Counseling

Three aspects of the component of counseling in nursing care of the long-term patient facing death are important. They are: planning care with the family, planning religious services for the patient, and planning with other health professions.

Though many families abnegate their responsibilities for a dying relative, other families want to do something in this final period. Planning what the family may do for the patient—how they can wipe a brow, or when they should call for a nurse—does much to help the dying patient and the family. The nurse helps the family work through their guilt feelings. Even in the best of relationships between patient and family guilt is a common reaction. It may be expressed in remarks such as, "I wish I had gone ahead and bought the color T.V. for her when she was still able to enjoy it."

The nurse should be alert to the patient's spiritual needs and should accept responsibility as a liaison between the patient, the family, and the requested clergy. If necessary, she should seek information in preparing for the clergy's arrival. There is a good deal of literature on religious beliefs and rituals and nursing responsibilities in specific religious observances.

It is the physician's responsibility to tell the patient and family if death is expected or imminent. The implementation of the doctor's decision to tell the patient and family, and the plan of care of the patient, is achieved through

Oh, yes! The doctor told the wife he couldn't last more than a day or two. She comes in and all she does is stand at the bedside and cry. So try to keep her out as much as possible.

The dying patient is very often a comatose, deeply sedated receptacle for numerous catheters, tubings, oxygen therapy, and various medications. The multiplicity of treatments, a common practice when death is imminent, complicates care. The skills of the nurse are taxed simply to maintain sufficient comfort and warmth from sheets and blankets for a restless patient and, at the same time, assure open draining of catheters.

The traditional setting for a dying patient is usually a darkened, warm, quiet room. However, some authorities now believe that the dying patient should have the same environment as any other patient, that is, a cheerful, bright, well-ventilated room. The latter seems much the better choice for a dying patient.

It is difficult to decide whether a private room or a ward is better for the dying patient. A private room affords him the quiet he may desire and need. It spares him the sight of other patients' pain and misery. It also allows for family visits any time during the night or day. A bed in a ward, on the other hand, provides contact with other patients, with ward personnel, and with diversional activities. The final choice should be made by the health team, who should weigh all the pros and cons of a given problem and try to judge which solution would be best for the patient. No matter what the decision is, the nurse should always maintain a close, physical contact with the patient. Communication, whether through holding the patient's hand, giving him a sip of water, straightening the top sheet, or talking to him, is of utmost importance.

Emotional care

How frequently do nurses provide only routine physical care, and fail to care for the patient as an individual! Emotional care for the dying patient involves two things. One is an understanding on the part of the nurse of her own views toward death—in other words, self-knowledge. The other is knowledge of the wide range of patient reactions, such as feelings of separation, of loss or of guilt. Comforting the patient, talking to him, orienting him, and even questioning him are some of the ways the nurse can maintain contact with the dying patient.

Self-knowledge was described by a nurse in the following words:

There was a taboo against expressing one's intimate feelings. It may be that the need for expression was greater in myself than in my patients. It seems to me important in such circumstances that we try to recognize our own inadequacies and seek such additional help and support for ourselves and our patients as may be necessary. This ultimately results in a better situation for us as individuals and in better nursing care which we can then give to patients.

Being adequately prepared to assist patients to meet death involves more than having a good professional education. A liberal arts background can supply information from literature, art, philosophy, psychology, and many other fields. The profession is responsible for preparing nurses to assist patients confronting death. This responsibility must first be recognized; it must then be expressed in sympathetic understanding, guidance, and supervision of nurses. Finally, it is the responsibility of the individual nurse to recognize and resolve her personal views toward death.

The other aspect of emotional care is understanding the wide range of patient reactions to death. Again, an example:

> One frail 80-year-old mother discussed her imminent death with me. She said her daughter did not want to hear her talk that way. Her one fear was that she might be dirty when the undertaker came for her. She wanted me, the visiting nurse, to prevent this. All the members of her family had stopped in to see her during the morning hours. During the early afternoon hours her strength rapidly failed. When I arrived and entered her room she recognized me and then seemed to relax. Her head rolled slowly to one side and from the corner of her mouth dark red fluid oozed and rolled down onto her chest. I wiped her face gently and, squeezing her hand, I said, "I'd better call your daughters."
> "We're here," came a voice from the doorway behind me. I turned to look into the eyes of the older daughter; the hand that I was holding grew limp, and a calm serenity spread across the mother's face. Cancer of the stomach had claimed another victim.
> This was my first experience with the outward evidence of hemorrhage. The old dying woman wanted to be clean. Did she have a premonition? I was able to comply with her request. She was clean, dressed in her favorite nightgown, and lying on a fresh bed when the morticians arrived.

Most dying patients want to talk about death. The nurse's usual reaction to this need is to establish emotional distance in order to block discussions about death. Emotional distance may be necessary for the emotional health of a patient's family and friends, but not listening to a patient who wants to talk about death is one of the most serious mistakes a nurse can make.

The authors' experience is the basis for the preceding sentence. A similar idea is expressed in a recent book by Dr.

Kübler-Ross in which she discusses the need for the dying patient to talk.[8] This book had such an impact that its ideas were discussed in such popular magazines as *Life*[9] and *Time*.[10]

Treatment

Prescribing treatment is the doctor's responsibility; following the doctor's orders with discretion is the nurse's responsibility. Yet treatments for the dying patient are beginning to have additional meaning. Current attacks upon the care of the dying patient center around the question, "What is life?" Because of medical advances, the health professions are able to prolong physical functions. But is this enough? "Medicated survival" is the term now used when only the physical functions are alive. Much has been written on this topic and on the patient's "right to die."

Dr. Vickery recently made world headlines following an address to the Congress on the hazards of retirement, which the Royal Society of Health held in Eastbourne, England. He stated that one of the cruelest hazards was "medicated survival." Dr. Vickery pleaded that old people beset with the pain, misery and indignity of intractable degenerative disease should be spared the prolongation of their suffering brought about by the use of wonder drugs and modern machine resuscitation. . . . doctors, nurses, and relatives caring for aged patients who are slowly and hopelessly dying from grave chronic illness are now faced with dilemmas unknown a generation ago. An added crisis like pneumonia, formerly known as "the old man's friend," can be promptly frustrated with an injection of antibiotic.[11]

Considerable rethinking should be done about the entire treatment pattern for the dying patient. While the most important function of treatment is to give comfort, this is often last considered. Medications should be given regularly and in amounts large enough to relieve pain. It close cooperation with the nurse and other professional workers. Coordination of all aspects of care contributes to maintaining the patient's dignity.

Economics

The economics of death are as important as the economics of long-term illness. Whether the patient is rich or poor, a financial worry may prevent him from dying with dignity. The man in his early forties needs to know that his will is written, that his estate will be handled as he desires, and that his family has a financially secure future. The nurse who helps a patient to contact his lawyer may be giving the patient the peace of mind that will allow him to die a peaceful death. Or the nurse may alleviate a poor widow's worry over a proper burial by telling her of inexpensive but dignified arrangements that can be made. The inward relief of the patient or relative can often be observed in a relaxation of facial muscles or lessened tension in the hand and fingers.

The nurse cares for the patient in a dollar-oriented society. Financial worries stay with the patient when he is admitted to the hospital; they cannot be closeted with his possessions. Awareness of how financial worries can affect a dying patient will increase the nurse's ability to give excellent care.

Complex correlations

An understanding of the factors that come into operation during the death of a patient can help the nurse give sensitive nursing care.

Hutschnecker[13] points out that the dying patient remains more or less true to his basic personality. The closeness of death may heighten or decrease some particular responses, but the patient is essentially the same person he was before his illness. The factors that precipitated the illness or which may have caused extension of the illness are still present.

The patient's attitude toward death directly influences his ability to meet it with dignity. These attitudes depend on his religious and cultural backgrounds, his philosophy, and his life experiences. Death can mean different things to different patients. It can represent:

    A teacher of transcendent truths that are incomprehensible during life
    A friend who brings an end to pain through peaceful sleep
    An adventure—a great, new oncoming experience
    The great destroyer who is to be fought to the bitter end
    A means of vengeance to force others to give more affection
    Escape from an unbearable situation to a new life
    A final narcissistic perfection, granting lasting and unchallenged importance to the individual
    A means of punishment and atonement[14]

Just as the patient's view of death influences his actions, so the nurse's view of death influences her ability to help the patient die with dignity. The nurse does not stop her care because the patient is dying—she uses her judgment to adapt her care to the change in needs. The more the nurse knows about the patient's pre-illness personality and the multiple relationships that existed during the earlier part of the illness, the broader is the base upon which she can make her professional judgment. True, such knowledge is not always available. But even when it is, nurses often do not use it.

DEATH, THE INEVITABLE: AN APPROACH

One nurse's care of a dying patient

It is not easy for a nurse to help a patient and his family meet death. One approach is through applying the eight components of long-term illness nursing. At times an hierarchy will form among the components; this blending and execution must be the basis of professional nursing care for dying patients. An example of how one nurse cared for a dying patient follows. Here is the blending of the varied dimensions of nursing care, the analysis of the situation, the synthesis which resulted in excellent patient care, and a well-stated description of professional nursing responsibilities.

About five years ago I cared for a patient whom we all knew was dying. He was 60 years old and had cancer throughout his body. He had a tracheotomy tube and a gastrostomy tube. His physical care became more and more complicated, as did his treatments.

He was unable to speak, but he could write notes to tell us what he wanted. In the last months of his illness his physical condition deteriorated rapidly, but his mind was alert to the end. The nurses called him a "difficult patient," but why shouldn't he have been difficult? He could not voice his wishes, and many times the nurses were in too much of a hurry to stop and read his notes. How very frustrated he must have been and how alone he must have felt. The last ten days of his life were spent in a private room. Then his actions became most difficult to cope with. He would have his light on to call the nurse almost constantly. He became so weak that his notes were illegible.

His wife lived about twenty miles away. She rarely visited him when he was first hospitalized, and not at all during the final stages of his illness.

I can imagine the panic the man must have felt—all alone in a room, no one to care about him, no one to understand him—knowing that he was dying and unable to make his wishes known. Small wonder that he would try to strike out at us and resist our care of him.

I was working nights, and had returned from my two nights off. He was particularly low. I made rounds to see him often, and left the small light on. He was awake when I went in around 2 a.m., and I sensed some kind of urgency. I remember how hard I tried to understand his weak gestures. The pencil kept falling from his fingers. I felt distressed. His eyes were begging, but I didn't know what he wanted. I knew he understood my words and I remember saying, "I want so much to understand you, Mr. Marros, but I just cannot." Then I helped him hold the pencil and told him to write just one word. With great effort he wrote a short word, and his hand fell back. I picked up the paper and tried to decipher the word. Suddenly I felt a chill at the back of my neck—the word was "die."

I could hardly say the word because I did not want to, but I did say it with a question mark. An expression of grateful relief came over his face; we had established contact. I could now ask questions, and he could respond with our finger signals of "yes" and "no." He wanted to see the doctor.

I called the nursing office and the night supervisor sent the doctor. The doctor was unable to communicate with him at all and saw no change in his condition. Both the night supervisor and the doctor said not to call his wife, and Mr. Marros did not request to see her. After the doctor left, Mr. Marros made no more attempts to communicate with me. I went in often, but he seemed to be sleeping. I turned him at regular intervals, the last time at 5 a.m. When I went in a few minutes later, he had died.

Somehow he had had a premonition of his death. I know he must have felt very alone. I wonder if he had resigned himself to death. He seemed peaceful at the end.

My own reaction was simple acceptance. I had known for many weeks that he would die. I felt a brief regret that he had to die, and then I knew that death was a release for him from all his suffering and frustration, and for that I could be almost relieved that he had died. My own religious beliefs gave me comfort. My regret was that his wife could not have been with him at the end (this was my need, not his or hers), but she may not have been able to provide any comfort to him because theirs was not a harmonious relationship. I wondered about her and whether she would have guilt feelings now that he was dead. Death is so final, and each person reacts differently to it. I feel that, as nurses, we do have responsibilities to patients and families at the time of death. I think death has to be faced and not evaded. Of course, it is hard. But we are nurses because we want to help people, and facing death is a time when people especially need understanding support. First of all, the nurse must have her own philosophy of life and death. We can then see that the patient's religious beliefs are followed, and support him in these beliefs. We can take good physical care of the patient and make him as comfortable as possible. We can simply be with him or with calm empathy express our feelings in words and actions. The family needs the same understanding support, and the desire of the patient and family to be together should be respected.

Death is inevitable and will one day come to each of us; death is an individual matter, and each family will meet it differently. With each patient and each family the nursing responsibility will vary. The nurse can do a great deal to help the patient, the family, her co-workers, and herself to meet death.

REFERENCES

1. Robb, Isabel Hampton, *Nursing Ethics*. Cleveland: E. C. Koeckert. 1909.
2. *Code for Nurses with Interpretative Statements*. New York: American Nurses' Association. 1968.
3. *Ibid*.

4. Mead, Margaret, The Right to Die. *Nursing Outlook. 16:* 10, Oct. 1968. pp. 20-21.
5. *Statistical Abstract of the United States.* Washington, D. C.: U.S. Bureau of the Census. 1969. p. 58.
6. *Op. cit.* p. 59.
7. Drummond, Eleanor E., and Jeanne E. Blumberg, Death and the Curriculum. *Journal of Nursing Education. 1:* 2, May-June 1962. pp. 21-28.
8. Kübler-Ross, Elisabeth, *On Death and Dying.* New York: Macmillan. 1969. 260 pp.
9. Wainright, Loudon, A Profound Lesson for the Living. *Life. 67:* 21, Nov. 21, 1969. pp. 36-43.
10. Out of Darkness. *Time,* Oct. 10, 1969. p. 60.
11. Vickery, Kenneth, O.A., The Right to Die. *This Week Magazine.* Aug. 17, 1969. pp. 4-5.
12. Saunders, Cicely, The Last Stages of Life. *American Journal of Nursing. 65:* 3, March 1965. pp. 70-75.
13. Hutschnecker, Arnold A., Personality Factors in Dying Patients, in *The Meaning of Death.* Herman Feifel, Ed. New York: McGraw-Hill. 1959. p. 237.
14. Feifel, Herman, Attitudes Toward Death in Some Normal and Mentally Ill Populations, in *The Meaning of Death.* Herman Feifel, Ed. New York: McGraw-Hill. 1959. pp. 126-127.

11 A CASE STUDY: A MODEL FOR NURSING CARE

The long-term patient has many nursing needs. Some are unique; some are universal. Some are simple; some are complex. Some are temporary; some are prolonged. All should be met with excellence of nursing care. But how? The care of the patient requires many things—a touch of tenderness, a giving spirit, physical exertion, a reservoir of knowledge and skills, and an understanding of nursing care. To fulfill these many requirements the nurse must have many resources.

By dividing the nursing care of the long-term patient into eight components, this book helps to mobilize the nurse's resources. The components can be blended, adapted, and interwoven into a program of specific nursing care. An example is the following case study which was reported to the authors by a senior baccalaureate student in the Registered Nurses' Program in the School of Nursing, University of California at Los Angeles.*

* The student, Marie Roberts, was enrolled in the Master's Program, School of Nursing, U.C.L.A., at the time this chapter was written. People, events, and situations in the case study were modified for purpose of its publication.

The story of this patient and her daughter includes some background information and the actual nursing care of the family. Each of the eight components of care is identified and discussed. Each component used by the nurse is not presented here in totality. Rather, one highlight of each component is discussed for the purpose of immediate comprehension. You will note that the sequence of components does not follow the sequence given in the preceding chapters. A specific patient situation determines the sequence and importance of any given component. (See page 3.)

Background information

Mrs. Grant, an 80-year-old woman who lived with her 50-year-old unmarried daughter, Miss Martha Grant, had been cared for by the visiting nurse (V.N.) for two years. The initial contact between the V.N. and Mrs. Grant occurred shortly after the insertion of a Neufeld nail for a fracture of the patient's left femur. She had had a peroneal nerve injury with a left foot drop after surgery. Her current diagnosis was generalized arteriosclerosis and malnutrition. Before the hip-nailing she had been well-developed and well-nourished; two years later she was thin, emaciated, and had pale conjunctivae and fingernails.

Mrs. Grant depended upon her daughter for the day-to-day care she required. The daughter had been progressively losing her eyesight during the past five years and could no longer work at her trade, which was operating a power sewing machine in a shirt factory.

The Grants looked to the V.N. for many services. Some progress of the family toward better health practices had been achieved. Mrs. Grant's muscles were free of contractures and her skin was in good condition.

The nursing care of the family

I prepared myself for the Grants by first reading their family record. Next, I discussed them, their nursing needs, and their nursing care plan with the V.N. who had been caring for them. When I knocked on the door of the Grants' apartment I was ready to give certain kinds of specific nursing care, anticipate certain nursing needs, alter the plan of care for the day, if necessary, and evaluate my care at a later date.

When I entered the home I talked briefly with the daughter and gradually approached Mrs. Grant. I smiled and talked quietly with her, told her who I was and what I wished to do for her. Throughout the visit I maintained a friendly interest in and respect for each of the Grants while I tried to provide good nursing care.

This is emotional support. These steps were taken to establish rapport and elicit confidence in the nurse and nursing procedures. The attitude of the nurse toward the elderly patient is a determining factor in her ability to gain the patient's cooperation and confidence. The patient needs affection, recognition, independence, and a sense of belonging and security. The patient also deserves respect and the rights and privileges to which she has been accustomed. By establishing a personal rapport with the patient through identifying herself and defining her role, the nurse encourages confidence, promotes continuity of care, and gives emotional support.

I gave Mrs. Grant a bedbath, changed her bed, and helped her to sit in a chair for a few minutes. At the same time I gathered information about her ambulation, diet, elimination, and the relationship between the mother and the daughter. Later, I recorded the substance of this one-hour encounter and set my goals for the next visit.

The second time I saw the Grants, the physician was making a home call at the same time. I was able to assist him in examining Mrs. Grant and talk with him about her care.

I pointed out to him the condition of her toenails and explained what I could and could not do about them. We all agreed that Mrs. Grant needed a chiropodist. The physician was pleased when I offered to call the Grants and give them the names of three chiropodists who made home calls; he was unaware of this service being available. Before the physician left I asked him to clarify the amount of ambulation he had prescribed for Mrs. Grant. Then, we planned for follow-up telephone contacts.

One type of counseling is the coordination of nursing with other services of the health team. By assisting the physician, the nurse can add to the care of the patient by contributing her observations and interpreting her responsibilities and limitations. The nurse needs a knowledge of other professional services available to the patient and methods of referral to those professional workers. Good communication enables the health team to maintain the patient's general condition and promote an optimum level of function.

After the physician left I talked about many things with the Grants, as I gave Mrs. Grant her bath. I massaged her back and explained why it was necessary and demonstrated how it was done. I left a pitcher of water beside Mrs. Grant's bed because I knew that her fluid intake was deplorably low. She had said that if she knew she could reach the water she'd drink it. I suggested that the daughter put fresh water in the pitcher each day.

The other type of counseling is engaging a family member in specific aspects of the nursing care of the patient. Generally, patients with peripheral vascular diseases should take larger amounts of fluids than the normal healthy person. In the home the nurse is seldom present twenty-four hours a day to offer fluids and insure a designated quantity of intake. Older people need to depend upon someone else to do and to remember to do many things. Therefore, a family member is the most logical person to help the older patient take sufficient fluids.

As I wrote up this visit I realized that I was just beginning to know the Grants and the many needs of the Grants.

The third time I saw the Grants I was glad to see them, and they gave me a hearty welcome. The chiropodist had come, and Mrs. Grant was very proud of her nails. While bathing Mrs. Grant I stressed the importance of elevating her head and chest while she was in bed and suggested ways of moving about in the bed. Then, with the help of the daughter, I assisted Mrs. Grant into a chair. I encouraged her to sit in the chair a little longer each day and to take a few more steps each day. I noticed that the shades in her room were drawn. She reluctantly agreed to have me raise them because she said the light from the window hurt her eyes. The daughter and I turned the bed so that Mrs. Grant would not be looking directly into the sunlight from her bed.

Attention to environmental characteristics of the patient's room is one aspect of physical care. A cheerful environment is essential to recovery and good mental health. A minor change in the location of furniture in the patient's room can contribute to the patient's comfort and to better control over the environment. Any change in the patient's room should be discussed with the patient and, ideally, agreed to by him. The older patient has more problems with change of any type, and the wise nurse is one who works with the patient to achieve acceptance of change.

When I inquired what Mrs. Grant usually ate and drank in a day, both she and her daughter told me. Their nursing care plan for the past two years had included the goal of a better diet. Yet only the breakfast seemed adequate. Mrs. Grant was very satisfied with her food, but her daughter was worried and said that meals were one of their biggest problems. She was very receptive to my suggestion that at my next visit we could spend some time talking about food, menus, cooking, and buying. (The record of this visit included a teaching plan for diet which extended into many future visits.)

On the fourth visit I came prepared to discuss diet with the Grants. They, too, were prepared. During the bath Mrs. Grant told me what she liked to eat, how she liked her food cooked, and when in her lifetime she'd eaten certain foods. She added that everything was just fine as it was right then. I talked with her about her current diet and said that she needed what she was eating. Then I added that there were a few foods which she needed and was not getting, and that she could add them a little at a time to her current diet. I went on to explain the effect her illness and current diet had upon her appearance because I knew she was concerned about her looks.

This is teaching. Older patients usually feel they are satisfied with their present diet regime. They cling to old habits. Usually protein, green leafy vegetables, and fruits are lacking in their diet, and they tend to live on a tea and toast regimen. But long-term patients need to be partners in their nursing care and, therefore, need to eat the foods that will prevent further illness and promote general health. To engage in the teaching-learning process, the nurse must try to find a point where the patient is amenable and likely to be motivated to change old habits.

Any diet change to unfamiliar foods or methods of cooking should be made gradually.

Later, the daughter told me about her problems with cooking and marketing and how set her mother was in her ways. I had selected three pamphlets to use because they had large print which could more easily be seen by the daughter. Miss Grant and I used these materials in evaluating their diet and seeing what foods were needed. I stressed to the daughter the importance of making only a few changes at a time, such as only one new food in a meal. (As I recorded the visit I knew that the test of my teaching would be whether or not the patient's diet did change.)

Mrs. Grant began the fifth visit by telling me during her bath that she was having many large, loose stools. I discovered that she was taking three five grain tablets of ferrous sulfate a day. I called the doctor, who discontinued the iron and said that he would plan to see the patient soon in order to determine future prescriptions.

Treatment is specified here. The nurse needs to know the reactions to any medication which the patient is taking. The local action of iron salts may cause a side effect. When iron is administered orally, it acts as an irritant and astringent which in the gastrointestinal tract may cause vomiting, nausea, constipation, or diarrhea. The nurse's responsibility is to notify the doctor when adverse reactions to a drug are developed by the patient.

This also gave me a good opportunity to pick up the diet instruction which I had begun. The daughter was most interested to learn about foods which affect the bowels. She told me with great pride that she had been able to add vegetable juice to their diet, and that her mother had liked it enough to ask her to do it again. Then she expressed concern over the food expenses as well as the expense of laundering the bed linens. I suggested that the next week we could sit down to look at their income and expenditures. She was eager for this and said that she'd get together her grocery slips, bills, and other receipts and try to figure out just what she was spending and where. (The visit and the plan for the next one were recorded, and budget assistance was included.)

As I knocked on the door of the Grant's apartment for the sixth time, I had with me some printed budget information. I noticed on the kitchen table little piles of grocery checks, papers with figures scrawled on them, various other receipts, and a couple of pencils. I followed the usual sequence of first giving Mrs. Grant her bath, assisting her into the chair, and making her bed. She said that she wasn't having the trouble with her bowels anymore and that she was feeling better. Then I sat down with the daughter and went over the budget information which I had brought. We looked at what she was spending on food, rent, and other items in relationship to the suggested proportions in the budget information. I advised her to make a shopping list, where and how to look for sales in the grocery store, and gave her some tips on what is and isn't a meat bargain. She was grateful for the assistance, and I felt that the time was well spent. Just my listening to the financial problems seemed helpful to the daughter.

Economics can be a very important component of the care of the long-term patient. The nurse must first recognize the economic problems. The nurse must be able to give basic budget assistance if needed. Families of older long-term patients will be able to give better care to them if they know how to spend their money wisely and have fewer financial worries. The nurse can do a great deal to help patients and families stretch what money they have.

Miss Grant also talked about no one's being available to stay with her mother when she had to go to the grocery or the laundermat, and about her difficulties in keeping the house straight and clean while caring for her mother. I suggested the Homemaker's Service and gave the daughter all of the information which she would need to contact them. I realized my misjudgment when she said she wasn't sure the Homemaker's Service was what she needed. She then proceeded to relate her concern for her mother, the fact that her mother needed more care than she could give her. When Mrs. Grant had been discharged three years ago, the daughter had been advised to send her mother to a rehabilitation convalescent home but had decided to care for her mother at home. Now she knew that she couldn't do it much longer.(I noted in my charting that day the daughter's growing awareness and acceptance of her inability to care for Mrs. Grant and the daughter's need for support in making the inevitable decision to hospitalize her mother.)

On the seventh visit the daughter greeted me at the door wholeheartedly before I had had a chance to knock. I bathed Mrs. Grant, then assisted her into the chair to sit there while I made her bed. I encouraged her to sit in the chair and walk a few more steps each day, telling her that she may even eventually walk to the bathroom to care for her own needs. When she walked, she demanded the assistance of her daughter but rejected help from me when I offered to walk on one side. I noticed two canes propped up against the wall across the room. I suggested she walk with one cane on one side and her daughter on the other. This she refused, too. When Mrs. Grant was back in bed I complimented her on walking a few steps, and she patted my face. I talked with the daughter about the use of a walker and found that Mrs. Grant had used one three years ago in the rehabilitation following the correction of her fracture. She had been reluctant to use it then but had tried it after the walker had been left in the room for a week for her to look at. If this was tried again, perhaps it would be successful again.

Each visit the daughter had discussed her partial blindness which she said was a gradually progressive impairment. I asked her when she had last had a complete physical examination. She couldn't remember definitely but said that it was years ago. I suggested that she should have a regular physical examination and that if finances were stopping her, she was eligible for care at a nearby county-financed clinic.

The nurse needs the knowledges of complex correlations, the body of knowledge in which statistical facts from diverse fields are related, to improve her patient care and aid the patient and her family in better maintenance of health. Here, two distinct statistical relationships are operative in the action of the nurse. One is that a familial history of a heart disease such as arteriosclerosis increases the likelihood that the disease will occur in succeeding generations. A second is that socio-economic factors play a large part in the delay of the diagnosis of a long-term illness, thereby decreasing the benefit which can result from treatment of the illness.

Before I charted this visit I consulted with the physical therapist in the agency about a walker for the patient. After a number of phone calls I found that no free walkers were available for loan at this time. However, I noted the telephone number of a community resource which seemed most likely in the near future to give to the Grants the walker they needed. (In my charting I noted to follow through on encouraging the daughter to obtain adequate medical care, to explore with her the idea of vocational rehabilitation, and to tell her about resources for the partially blind in the community.)

The eighth and last time I cared for the Grants I felt a sense of loss, knowing it would be my last visit. As I was bathing Mrs. Grant I noticed that her skin was in good condition but that she'd developed a small reddened area over the coccyx.

Observation is of utmost importance in the care of long-term patients who spend most of their time in bed. The skin of the elderly patient requires special attention. Pressure areas occur where bony prominences are subject to local irritation—the body weight being constantly upon the coccyx of a person lying on her back in bed twenty-four hours a day. Decubitus ulcers begin with a reddened spot in the skin, which is warm to the touch and sometimes tender to the patient. The nurse needs to use her sense of sight and touch in detecting the initial stages of a decubitus ulcer.

I showed the spot to the daughter and suggested that she massage the area at least twice a day and make sure that her mother change her position in bed frequently. This gave me an opportunity to discuss again with both of them the importance of Mrs. Grant's getting out of bed. In vain, I tried to interest Mrs. Grant in finding a way to keep her stockings up without garters which were constricting the vessels of her legs. She said she'd always worn stockings with garters and that she intended to continue to do so. I turned my attention to the foot board which Mrs. Grant had used for two years. I noticed that the bedding was over the foot board and praised both the Grants for it. They laughed. Proper bedmaking with a foot board had taken four months to accomplish and was a big achievement. The daughter asked me to sit down at our usual place, the kitchen table, and talk about the permanent care of her mother and what she'd do when her mother was in a home. She had been doing a lot of thinking and just wanted to talk about it. Before I left I told the Grants that this was my last visit and that they should expect Mrs. Rogers next time.

At the office I charted my last visit. Then, I discussed the care I had given the Grants with Mrs. Rogers, the V.N. who would continue their nursing care.

The nursing care of the Grants was accomplished through one-hour nurse-patient contacts per week. This is a very short time considering the long-term patient's need for nursing care. The nursing care of the Grants would, of course, have been different if another nurse had acted in the same situation. Whatever the care would have been, this nursing care cited was excellent.

The case study of the Grants was analyzed according to

the eight components of the care of the long-term patient. Only one action of the nurse was discussed for each of these vital components. It was shown that the components varied in time and that the priority of the eight components shifted as the needs of the patient changed. Flexibility and adaptability are necessary in the application of nursing knowledge and skills. It is the conscious interweaving of the components to meet individual differences and changing needs that achieves excellence in the nursing care of the long-term patient.

INDEX

Air pollution, 105
Allergy, 65
Ambulation, transition to, 38
American Cancer Society, 91
Anemia, 20
Antidepressant drugs, 100-101
Arterial disease, diet and salt intake, 105
Arteriosclerotic heart disease, 98
Arthritis, 13, 24
  care of hand, 38
  rheumatoid, 23
Atherosclerosis
  diet, 104-105
  hypertension in, 105

Bathing, 35-36
  frequency of, 35
  special equipment, 35
Bed and bedding, 32
Bedpan, use of, 34
Benedict Qualitative Test, 15
Bladder rehabilitation, 34-35
Bodily protection, 31-32
Body image and role, 52-53
Boredom, 51
Bowel rehabilitation, 34-35
Bowel control in cerebrovascular incidents, 38
Budgeting, 12
  teaching of, 92

Bureau of Public Assistance, 12, 91

Cancer, 13
Cardiovascular mortality rates, factors in, 104
Case history material, persons used by, 18-19
Catheters, use of, 34
Cerebrovascular incident
  bed and equipment needed, 28
  control of bladder and bowels, 38
Cholesterol level, effect of stress, 97
Chronic diseases, 2, 13, 97
  definition, 2
  feeling of helplessness, 97
  long-term patients with, 2
  nursing, 2
Clothing, 31-32
Cobalt therapy, reactions to, 64-65
Code for Nurses With Interpretative Statements, 107-108
Communications
  necessity for, 24
  verbal and non-verbal, 25, 41-44
Community resources, 75-76
Complex correlations, 12-13, 95-106
  case history, 82
  in diet and patient aid, 133-134
  dying patients, 119-120
  ethnic factors, 98, 103

nurse's approach to multiple diseases, 101-102
presence of more than one disease, 99-100
socio-economic factors, 102-105
totality of body and mind, 98-99
Counseling, 78-86
case history, 128-129
dying patients, 118-119
the family, 21
patient and family, 78-86
working with the health team, 11,28
Crutches, training for, 38

Death, 107-124
causes in chronic conditions, 109
Code for Nurses with Interpretive Statements, 107-108
incidents cited by nurses, 109-111
leading causes, 108-109
meaning of to different patients, 120
new definition, 108
nurse's feelings concerning, 47
nurse's views of, 120
unexpected, 111-112
in Western culture, 107
Depression, 52
Diabetes, 13,20
Dietician, reliance on nurse's observations, 16
Diet planning, 12
Diseases
correlations in, 96-98
economic factors in, 103-104
ethnic factors, 96
familial factors, 96-97
familial history, 102
socio-economic factor, 96-97
stress factor, 97
Diuretic therapy, 65
Drainage bag, acceptance of, 73
Draping during examination, 31
Drugs, see also Medication
keeping up with new, 20, 59

ordering by generic name, 93
reporting toxic reactions to, 25
sources of information, 62
toxic reactions, 20
Dying patients, 107-136
case history, 121-123
complex correlations, 119-120
counseling, 118-119
economics, 119
emotional care, 114-116
environment, 113
helping the family, 118
medication, 117
need to discuss death, 115-116
observations, 111-112
physical care, 112-113
responsibilities of nurse, 111-123
spiritual needs, 118
teaching, 117-118
treatment, 116-117

Economic level, effect of, 98
Economics of long-term illness, 87-94
budget planning, 12, 92, 132
case history, 82, 87-88
Commission on Chronic Illness, 89
of disability, 11-12
of dying patients, 119
increased medical costs, reasons for, 89
medicare, 89
nurse's attitude, 90
nurse's responsibilities, 89, 91
over 65, Public Law 89-97, 89
patient's reticence to discuss financial problems, 90
referral to other agencies, 90-91
sources of help, 88-89
Emotional support, 40-56
body language, 41-42
case history, 81
in change in body image and role, 52-53
during depression, 52

INDEX

of dying patients, 114-116
listening to patient, 42-44, 50
in nurse-patient relationship, 8-9
nursing responsibility, 40-44
social amenities and spiritual support, 53-54
use of touch, 40-42
Enemas, use of, 34
Environment of patient, 22-23, 30-31, 129
Equipment
improvising, 12, 92
learning use of new, 65-66
Esalen, 41
Ethnic origins, effect on learning, 72-73
Exercises and exercising, 36-37
in the bath, 36
handbooks, 36
for mastectomy, 36
need for, 37
nurse's responsibilities, 36-37
prescribed by doctor, 36

Family
counseling, 11, 21, 78-79
disability, economics of, 11-12
home environment for patient, 23, 30-31
teaching, 80-82
in open-heart surgery, 67
Fears of patient, 49-52
of helplessness, 50-51
of loss of body-part, 51-52
sensitivity to pain and, 50
Feeding, 32-33
attitudes toward food, 32-33
need for encouragement, 33
need to eat well in certain diseases, 20
nurse's responsibilities, 33
self-feeding, 33
tube-feeding, 33
Ferrous sulfate, 131

Financial problems, see also Economics
in death, 119
sources of assistance, 12
Fluids, need for, 128

Germ theory, 12-13
inadequacy of, 105

Hair, care of, 29, 35
Health team
focus, 84
need for conferences, 83-84
patient's relationship with, 21
working relationships, 84-86

Heart disease, 13
effect of crowding, 103
Heart failure, congestive, 20
Helplessness, 51
Help Yourself to Recovery, 36
Hemorrhage, necessity for immediate report, 24
Hospital
adjusting to, 73
role of patient, 74
Hypertension, associated with atherosclerosis, 105

Independence, developing in patient, 29
Indigency, 104
Iron, 131
Isoniazid, 63

Laboratory tests, management, 92
Leg and foot, supporting and conditioning, 38
Listening With the Third Ear, 71
Loneliness, 51
Long-term illness, effect on patient, 9
Long-term patient
changes in, reviewing and re-

porting, 25
definition, 1-2
environment, 22-23
knowledge they require, 73-75
needs, 2
nursing needs, 125
observations of, 27

Mantoux test, 60
Mastectomy, 25
    exercises for, 36
Medicaid, 12
Medical students, patient's reaction to, 22
Medicare, 89
Medicated survival, 116
Medication, for dying patients, 117
Monoamine oxidase inhibiting drugs, 20
Motivation, 38-39
Multiple sclerosis, 23
    environmental needs, 30

Nails, care of, 35
Nursing care
    a case study, 125-136
    delegation of responsibilities, 80-82
    physical care, 8, 28-39
    skills needed, 5-7
Nurse-patient relationship, 2-8
    body language and use of touch, 40-42
    collector relationship, 18-19
    concern for costs, 93
    depression, 52
    discussing financial problems, 90
    emotional support, 8-9, 40-56
    explaining medications, 63-64
    financial problems, 11-12
    gaining patient's confidence, 127
    how nurse's attitudes effect patient, 68
    interviewer, 18
    learning from patient, 58-59
    listening to patient, 42-44, 50
    model of nursing care, 5
    explanation of model, 3-7
    need for close contact, 18
    observation
        need for, 7-8
        need for a system, 19
    participant relationships, 19
    patient's need to verbalize, 50
    selection of hospital room, 30
    spectator relationship, 18
    teaching patient about his illness, 74-75

Nurses
    ability to listen, 42-44
    correlations, recognition of, 13
    developing insights, 48
    dietician's need for nurse's observations, 16
    economic responsibilities to patient and his family, 12
    the family, working with, 11
    feelings, 46-47
        about long-term patient, 47
    greeting new patient, 53
    handling new types of equipment, 65-66
    keeping up with new drugs and techniques, 10, 75
    knowledge required, 59-60
    listening to patient, 70-71
    need for change, 47-48
    observation, 15-27
        of patient's attitude toward hospital personnel and his family, 22
        of patient's physical abilities, 15
    perception of family relationships, 15
    physician's need for her observations, 15
    questions for nurse to ask and answer, 61-66
    referral responsibilities, 90-91
    reports, 24, 64

INDEX

responsibilities
  additional, 80-82
  in death, 111-123
  for effect of drugs, 20
  extent of, 27
  professional, 61-66
  in sphere of economics, 89-90
self-analysis, 44-47
self-knowledge, 8-9, 44-49, 69, 114
sensitivity, 16-17
sixth sense, need for, 16-17
social worker's need for her observations, 15
study, need for, 96
teaching activities, 10-11, 67-77
teaching the patient, 58, 68-69
understanding the patient, 9
views of death, 120
working with the health team, 11, 21

Observation, 15-27
  attitudes of patient towards others, 22
  case history, 80
  communicating, 24-27
  of dying patient, 111-112
  environment of patient, 22-23, 30-31, 129
  keeping records, 26-27
  need for, 7
  of reaction to drugs, 19-20
  of reactions to treatment, 64-66
Old Age Survivors Insurance, 12
Oral hygiene, 36
Orinase, in combination with fulfinamide, 20
Ornade, 63
Osteoporosis, 64

Parenteral preparations, 63
Parkinson's disease, 24
Pharmacists, 62
Phenobarbitol, 100
Physical care, 28-39
  bed and bedding, 28

bodily care, 8, 28-29, 31, 35, 37, 112-113
bodily protection, 28
case history, 81
dying patient, 112-113
environmental control, 30
hair, 29
need for, 37
Physicians, reliance on nurse's observations, 15
Pohl, Margaret, *The Teaching Function of the Nursing Practitioner*, 67
Population, effect of density, 103
Poverty, long-term illness and, 11-12
Powdered milk, use of, 92
Psychosomatic diseases, correlations, 96

Rauwolfia preparations, reactions to, 64
Records, importance of, 26-27
Referral
  nurse's responsibilities, 90-91
  systems, 76
Reik, Theodor, *Listening With the Third Ear*, 71
Religious practices, 54
Respiratory disease and air polution, 105
Rheumatoid arthritis, 97
Right to die, 116

Sixth sense, 16-17
Skin, care of in bedridden patients, 134
Smoking, 97, 105
Social Agencies, Directory of, 76
Social relationships of patients, 21
Social workers, need for nurse's observations, 15
Spiritual support, 53-54
Spiritual needs of dying patients, 118
Steroid therapy, reactions to, 64
Stress, 101-102
Strike Back at Arthritis, 36
Strike Back at Stroke, 58

Stroke, 57-58
Support and positioning, 37-39
  for an arthritic hand, 38
  leg and foot, 38
  motivations for independence, 38-39
  to promote muscular control, 37-38
Teaching, 67-77
  the family, 80-82
Teaching the patient, 10-11, 58, 67-77
  attention span of patient, 72
  budgeting, 92
  case history, 80-81
  to change behavior, 69
  content, 70-73
  about diet, 130
  dying patients, 117-118
  effect of ethnic origins, 72-73
  general health measures, 76
  guidelines, 70
  length of sessions, 72
  listening and observing, importance of, 70-71
  long-term patient about his illness, 68
  materials, 70
  method, 70, 72
  in open-heart surgery, 67
  planning, 67-68
  process recording, 69
  questions, 70, 71
  self-help, 67-68, 74-75
  use of equipment, 92
The Teaching Function of the Nursing Practitioner, 67
Teeth, care of, 36

Thiazide diuretic, in combination with digitalis, 20
Time, meaning of to patients, 23-24
Time test, 60
Toileting, 33-35
  bedpan, 34
  bowel and bladder rehabilitation, 34-35
  catheters, 34
  constipation and diarrhea, 33-34
  enemas, 34
Treatment, 57-66
  analysis in long-term illness, 59
  case history, 81-82
  complexities, 9-10
  definition, 57
  diagnostic procedures, 9
  dosage and administration, 9
  of dying patients, 116-117
  economic aspects, 57
  keeping up with current, 10, 59-60
  mechanics of, 58
  questions to be asked and answered, 61-62
  therapeutic procedures, 9
Tuberculosis, 97
  arrested, 15
  economic factors in, 98
  Kuwaiti children, vs. Lebanese, reactions to tuberculin, 98
  stress, effect of, 97

Workman's Compensation, 12

X-ray, reactions to, 64-65